SIMPLY
Beautiful

SIMPLY
Beautiful

HEAD-TO-TOE
QUICK TIPS AND PRO TRICKS
FOR LOOKING GREAT
IN NO TIME FLAT

Linda Stasi

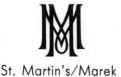

St. Martin's/Marek

Photo credits

Page 1:—Hair: *Jeffrey McDonald* for YVES CLAUDE HAIR; Color: *Michael Stinchcomb* for YVES CLAUDE HAIR; Photography: *Nancy DePra;* Makeup: *Diane Matthews;* Stylist: *Mark Donofrio*

Page 33:—Courtesy of Chanel, Inc.

Page 74:—Courtesy of Danskin, Inc.

Page 118:—Photograph by *Stephen Congiusta, Weight Watchers* magazine

Pages 25, 27, 35, 45, 48, 52, 76, 83, 87, 88, 90, 93, 95, 101, and 103:—Hair and Makeup: *Dale Susan Darmante;* Model: *Lisa Martin;* Photography: *Walt Denson*

Design by Laura Hammond

Library of Congress Cataloging in Publication Data
Stasi, Linda.
    Simply beautiful.
    1. Beauty, Personal.   2. Women—Health and hygiene.
I. Title.
RA778.S796   1983   646.7   82–19156
ISBN 0–312–72591–4 (pbk.)

First Edition
10 9 8 7 6 5 4 3 2 1

DEDICATION

*For my little beauty—my daughter Jessica
and for my Mom*

Contents

3. BODY SHOP

4. HAND AND FOOT NOTES

5. BEFORE WE SAY GOODBYE

Acknowledgments

Thank You:
Julia Coopersmith, the world's best agent and most patient friend;
someone who's never too tired to let me whine and dine. Pat Con-
way, for helping to turn a mountain of scripts into a semblance of
order and a mountain of typed pages. Joyce Engelson, my editor, for
believing, and reading and believing. Clarice Turnbull for typing and
sorting, and typing and sorting. Stephen Auerbach for giving me a
place in which to do it all, and a shoulder. Deborah Daly, St.
Martin's art director, for her wonderful talent. And for everyone
whose name appears in this book for giving freely of their time
. . . and their secrets.

Introduction

There are books about beauty and books about breasts. Some books deal strictly with your bottom, while others tell you how to dress your way to the top. Some of these books are for men, some are for women, some for teens. But this book is filled with quick, inexpensive top-to-toe tips for everyone.

And that's what this book is all about: looking like a million for pennies. In it, you'll find ways to make your own facials, hair conditioners, and even makeups that would normally cost a bundle. And you'll also find quick tests that will help you size up the skin you're in, the shape you take, and even the ways to correct both. You'll also discover little known facts that can turn you into an authority on . . . yourself. You'll learn how to achieve the look you've always wanted from the very people who have created the unique "looks" of some of the world's most famous faces . . . and bodies. Who are some of these people? Makeup and hair designers, fashion and beauty editors, top models, doctors, nutritionists, and exercise experts, for starters. And there's more.

But these pages are designed for fun. Let's face it, no one has ever died from wearing the wrong hair-do (although we've all felt that we could have died of embarrassment at some point when our latest "do" just didn't).

Looking good and feeling terrific is fun. All you need is the key that will unlock the look that you want . . . and the one that's right for you. So read on. Chances are you'll not only find the solutions to your dilemmas but you'll enjoy yourself as well. So let's get started making you over from head to foot . . . without breaking your bank.

SIMPLY
Beautiful

1
Hair Do's
And Don'ts

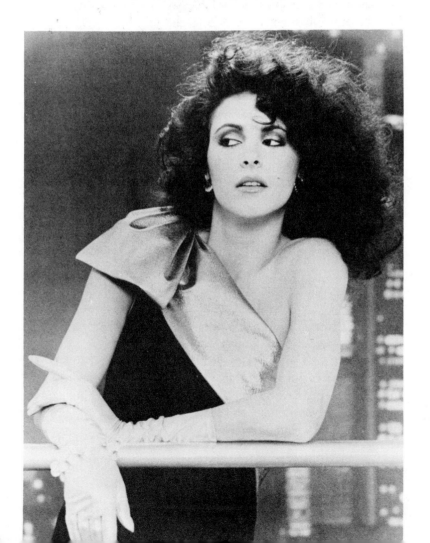

FACTS, FALLACIES, AND FOLLICLES

You can grow it, show it and blow it, and still not know it very well. If you've ever wondered how much of what you've heard about your hair is fact and how much is fable, you may be surprised to learn that it's probably a good chunk of each.

GROW IT

Because hair is sexy, it's always been surrounded both by lust and legend. Take Samson, for example. If you believe that his tale of woe has no basis in fact, you've probably never gotten a truly rotten haircut before a really important event. (A truly rotten haircut usually includes one-inch Mamie Eisenhower bangs.) Let's face it, how powerful can you feel when you know in your heart that you look like your Aunt Cecelia when she had the poodle cut?

KNOW IT!

But, thankfully, even the worst haircut—unlike a pair of too-short pants—grows back. In fact, your hair actually grows at the rate of about one-half inch per month. Fall-out, however, is also very rapid. Estimates put the average hair loss at anywhere between 50 and 150 hairs per day! So don't panic if you think that there are too many hairs on your pillow, and too few on your head. It's probably just the normal shedding process.

But what about the shape it takes? Did you ever wonder—when you were little—why you were cursed with straight hair while your best friend (or your brother) got the naturally wavy locks?

That's because all hair is made up of keratin—a protein. Your hair also has roots, follicles, and hair shafts or strands. The follicle is what shapes the hair strand. If you have round strands you will have straight hair, oval strands produce wavy hair, and flat strands produce curly or frizzy hair. If you are also lucky enough to have "thick" hair, it means that you have many hair roots which are placed closely together on the scalp.

SHOW IT

Hair color is actually as trendy as style. How many platinum blondes, for example, do you see walking around these days? Not a whole lot. Still blondes will always be equated with glamour . . . and fun. But if blondes do have more fun, perhaps it's because they have more hair. Natural blondes, of which there are three known to be living (all in Denmark, eating yogurt), have about 140,000 hairs per head (that figure, of course, has nothing to do with born-again-and-again blondes). Brunettes have about 115,000, and redheads have only about 80,000 strands per head.

BLOW IT!

Remember when you spent a good deal of your life in curlers and a hairnet? Now if you spend it maneuvering a blow dryer around, the first thing you should know is that you shouldn't. The second thing you should know is how you can stop. The third and most important thing? How you can make your hair look like a million for pennies!

PROFESSIONAL TRICKS, TIPS, AND RECIPES . . . THE KIND THAT ONLY YOUR HAIRDRESSER KNOWS FOR SURE AND SURELY WON'T *TELL* YOU!

SOLUTIONS, TESTS, TIPS, AND TRICKS TO COMBAT EVEN THE WORST HAIR DILEMMAS

SUGA'S TEST FOR TEXTURE . . .

World-famous hairdresser, Suga, gave me this tip when he appeared on my program:

Shampoo and towel dry your hair. In a normally heated room, fine hair should air dry naturally in 15 to 20 minutes; medium hair in 30 to 45 minutes; and coarse hair will take more than 45 minutes. If you can't stand the suspense of not knowing immediately, a hand-held blower will dry fine hair in 5 to 8 minutes; medium in 8 to 15 minutes, and coarse hair in 15 minutes or longer. The exceptions, of course, are very long or very short hair.

DANDRUFF AND OTHER UNPLEASANT FACTS OF LIFELESS HAIR

Did you also know that if you've got hair, chances are you'll develop dandruff at some point in your life? Dandruff is *not* a disease. It *is* the natural shedding of dead cells from the scalp.

GETTING CONTROL

To keep the snowstorm off of your shoulders and under control:

• Try brushing your hair rigorously before you shampoo, with a soft sparkling clean brush.
• Use a good therapeutic tar-based shampoo, like *Polytar*™ from Stiefel Laboratories, Inc., and gently massage your scalp

with your fingertips or knuckles (don't scratch it with your nails).
• Rinse well and rinse again because residual shampoo can dry, flake, and itch your scalp.
• A cool final rinse will help to close up the pores.

A MANE FOR ALL SEASONS

Dandruff is frequently seasonal. You may, for example, find that your personal snowstorm kicks up more in winter. No, it's not because it's cold outside: it's the opposite. Overheated rooms with forced hot-air heating, or rooms that are poorly ventilated can cause your scalp to dry out in much the same way that those same conditions cause your skin to dry out—*so turn down the heat!*

SEBORRHEA, YOU SAY?

Now that you know how to control normal dandruff, you might find that your condition is a more complex personality. In that case it just might be seborrhea. While seborrhea *is* more serious, it can usually be controlled. *Here's how:*

• Keep your hair well-brushed every day to keep the flakes at bay.
• Wet your hair, apply a medicated tar-based shampoo, and leave it on for 3 to 5 minutes.
• Then rinse, relather, and rinse again until your hair is squeaky clean.

And make sure that you keep your skin as well-washed as your hair because the flakes can cause complexion problems as well.

PEACH FUZZ AND CREAM COMPLEXION

It's not just the hair on your head that can cause problems on your face, it's also the peach fuzz that grows along your jawline, according to Janet Sartin, world-famous skin care authority. The peach fuzz along your hairline has a tendency to clog pores and cause blemishes when mixed with the oil from your hair. So if you've got oily hair be sure to wash it every day or every other day at the very least. If possible, keep your hair off your face, too.

WELL-OILED

Is the glorious shine in your hair coming from too much oil rather than too much health? (I know that mine's too oily when I go for a dramatic swing of the hair and it swings like a solid concrete mass.) If you'd rather avoid going to extremes and possibly hurting someone with your hair, try shampooing in this manner:

- Apply shampoo to your hair *before* you wet it.
- Massage the shampoo into your dry hair and scalp to help break down excess oil buildup.
- Slowly add water, then shampoo, rinse, relather and rinse well.
- If you use conditioner, use it sparingly. Too much conditioner can't be absorbed by the hair, and can leave a greasy coating. You want a small amount on the inside, not globs on the outside.

TAKING YOUR HAIR TO THE CLEANERS
(What Type and How to Wash It)

Dry Hair—Your scalp simply isn't producing enough oil, so use a cream or lotion shampoo with lots of conditioner to replace lost oil.

Oily Hair—It tends to hold dirt, so clean it with a shampoo that has a high detergent level.

Normal Hair—Baby shampoos or *Silkience™ Shampoo* from Gillette are great and very mild especially if you shampoo every day.

FIGHTING THE FRIZZIES

Hair gone haywire? Then try this trick: Spray a tissue with hair spray and smooth it over the flyaway hairs to bring them back down to earth.

SHOCK WAVES

If your hair seems to have enough electricity to power the city of Detroit on any given day try any of these quick tricks:

- Spray your hairbrush with conditioning hair spray, and brush lightly over the top hairs.
- Take extra care when you wash your hair. Massage the scalp gently, don't scrub or scratch.
- Spray your hairbrush lightly with an antistatic (laundry) product before you style.
- Stay away from blow dryers or use only when necessary.
- Ditto for curling irons and hot curlers.
- Keep your hair well-moisturized with weekly or semimonthly hot oil treatments. (See *It's a Natural,* page 9.)
- Use a cream rinse after each shampoo.
- Use a dab of cream or water each time you style.

Let's face it, only the Bride of Frankenstein ever got away with exploding hair, and that was because she'd probably have eaten the foot of the first person who complained.

TO MAKE LESS LOOK LIKE MORE

Do you love your hair? (All twelve strands of it?) Well, even if you never could *grow* a thick head of hair, at least you can fake a thick head of hair. *Here's how:* Bend over from the waist and brush from the nape of your neck forward. Then spray lightly with hair spray, stand back up and flip your hair back. Shake your hair vigorously and finger-comb or lightly brush into place.

BONUS TIPS AND TRICKS FOR THIN HAIR

• Get a blunt cut. Thin hair looks fuller when it's cut this way.
• Use a mixture of two conditioners, one that contains protein and one, moisturizer. Comb the mixture through your hair and secure it with a clip. Rinse it out after 30 minutes.

GET INTO CONDITION

When the summer sun leaves your body sleek and gorgeous and your hair dried-out and crummy, try hairdresser, Vincent Bruce's, secret hot pack for hair. *Here's how:* Wash your hair before you leave for the beach or pool. Comb a high-protein conditioner directly into wet hair. If your hair is long, pull it back into a chignon and hold it in place with bright combs. Short hair? Slick it back into a head-hugging style. The heat from the sun will activate the conditioner to work as a hot cap. When you get back home, simply shampoo your hair till it squeaks.

Bonus: The conditioner also coats your hair, creating a sunscreen for it. So, you can skip the hat or scarf.

KEEPING COMBS IN PLACE

If keeping hair combs and barrettes in place is as much of a nuisance to you as letting your hair fall into your eyes, spray the section of your hair where you'll be inserting the ornament with hair spray. Insert the comb and spray again. Voilà! Hair to stay. Gillette's New Mink Difference™ hair spray is good for this because it leaves you with soft natural-looking hair, instead of a helmet.

HUMIDITY AND THE HAIR

If summer is frizzy hair season for you, you'll want to, know why it happens and what you can do about it. First, summer humidity isn't all bad, in fact, it's great . . . for your hair. It helps to moisturize it and keep it in good condition. However, as moisture enters the hair shaft it causes your natural curl to appear. So be sure to use a cream rinse after shampooing.

CURL CONTROL

When you blow your hair:

- Use the biggest round hair brush you can find. There's one marvelous one from *Spornett*™ that is made of natural boar bristles, and is about 3 inches in diameter. It will help keep you straight for hours!
- A good haircut, too, can help by giving you wash-and-wear hair.
- Finally, don't try to force your hair to go straight *every* day, because in the end, it's a losing battle. (Besides, lots of curls are terrific in the summer, especially with casual skimpy clothes.)

If your hair reaches steel wool proportions you may be holding the hair blower too close or using a shampoo that's too harsh. Get professional advice and get the ends trimmed frequently.

Try an anticurl hairdo such as a chignon or ponytail. Just be sure to leave a little slack in the back . . . pulling too tightly on your hair can cause hairline breakage.

IT'S A NATURAL

RECIPES FOR MAKING GREAT HAIR PRODUCTS WITH INGREDIENTS YOU'LL FIND RIGHT AROUND YOUR KITCHEN

HAIR TEA-ZING
(All Hair Types)

Ingredients:
5 bags of chamomile tea

Tea, especially chamomile tea, makes a super hair rinse which will give your hair so much shine, you'll look like you've got the light on in your head!

Here's how: Just brew a pot of chamomile tea and chill it overnight in the fridge. Then after you've shampooed and rinsed your hair very well, pour a pitcher of the chilled tea through your hair. Then just watch out for the shining!

GIVE YOUR HEAD THE COLD SHOULDER

If you don't have time to brew the tea, remember that it's a good idea always to use cold water . . . straight from the tap, for free, or from a mineral water bottle—for a fee . . . as a final hair rinse. Cold water closes up the hair cuticles, which gives your hair electric light shine . . . if you can stand the shock.

DORIS MC MILLON'S GO SOAK YOUR HEAD HAIR CONDITIONER
(For Normal, Dry, and/or Damaged Hair)

Ingredients:
½–1 cup olive oil

As a top New York City television reporter, Doris McMillon needs to have shining, well-managed hair, so she gives her head this soak every other week or so.

Heat about ½ to 1 cup of olive oil till just warm. How much you use depends on the length of your hair. Massage the warmed oil into your hair and scalp and then cover your hair with clear plastic wrap. (Yes, you will look like a salad in a cafeteria.) Leave the oil on your hair at least an hour—or sit under a hood type hair dryer, set on low for 20 minutes. Then just shampoo and rinse until your hair is very clean.

RAPHAEL'S EGG-HEAD CONDITIONER
(Adds Body to Any Hair Type)

Ingredients:
½ cup lemon juice
1 egg separated
1 cup water

What, besides pudding, do you get if you mix an egg yolk with lemon? A super, and very inexpensive hair conditioner! This one was developed by one of New York's best hairdressers, Raphael Santa Rosa.

Shampoo your hair once, and apply a lightly beaten egg yolk. Massage it in and all around your hair. After 5 minutes, rinse well with hot water. Then rinse with cooler water until your hair is really clean. Finally pour a bowl of lemon juice and water through your hair as a final rinse.

AVOCADO AFFICIONADO
(For Dry, Lifeless Hair)

Ingredients:
½ avocado
1 well-beaten egg

Mash the avocado half and mix it with a beaten egg. Massage the mixture into your hair and scalp, and then cover your head with a dry towel. (This is not to keep passersby from dunking crackers into your head. It's to hold the conditioner.) Let it sit for 15 minutes and follow up with your regular shampoo.

Bonus Tips: Mix some of the mashed avocado into your shampoo for extra nourishment; plant the pit and grow your own conditioners at home!

MADEMOISELLE MAGAZINE'S HENNA HIGHLIGHTER
(Normal, Oily Hair)

Ingredients:
1 package neutral henna
2 eggs
1 summer day

Here's *Mademoiselle*'s recipe for super shine and body. Mix together one package of neutral powdered henna with water, as indicated on package, in a nonmetallic container. Add two eggs to form a thick paste. Then coat your hair, from the roots to the ends, by gently rubbing the mixture into your hair. Step into the sun and let the mixture "cook" for about 20 to 30 minutes. Shampoo and rinse thoroughly.

CREATE AN OIL SHORTAGE HAIR RINSE
(For Oily Hair)

Ingredients:
1 package of neutral henna

Try this ancient beauty secret to keep the oil level in your hair down to a minimum.

Shampoo as usual and rinse thoroughly. Then mix a package of neutral henna with warm water and pour the mixture through your hair. Leave on for an hour and rinse off. Then shampoo and style as usual. The henna will remove most of the excess acid and oil, so your hair strands will actually lie flatter, making it more difficult for residue oil to collect.

A word of caution: While henna is wonderful, terrific, and gorgeous for your hair, it can also cause it to dry out if you become overly enthusiastic. It's unhealthy to henna your hair more than once every 3 months or so.

MORE WAYS TO CREATE AN OIL SHORTAGE IN YOUR HAIR
(For Oily Hair)

Ingredients:
skim milk
1 teaspoon of salt

Dissolve salt in skim milk, and rub it into your scalp. Don't rinse it out, just let your hair dry. Shampoo and rinse thoroughly after about an hour.

YUMMY YOGURT HAIR CONDITIONER
(All Hair Types)

Ingredients:
1 beaten egg
½ cup plain yogurt

If the health food wave has stirred your guilt because you hate yogurt and love preservative-filled hot dogs, alleviate your conscience by nourishing your hair with yogurt.

Mix the yogurt and egg together. Shampoo and towel-dry your hair and comb the yogurt mixture through. Leave it on for 30 to 40 minutes and rinse thoroughly with warm water. Follow up with the lemon and water rinse described earlier. Voilà! Well-fed hair!

HAIR SETTING LOTIONS THAT YOU'LL FIND ONLY IN YOUR REFRIGERATOR AND OTHER INCONSPICUOUS PLACES

I'm *afraid* that it looks as though we may be in for a revival of the hair do. Be prepared! and don't be surprised if you find yourself fantasizing about teasing combs before the year is out! Here, to get you into the swing of hair that doesn't, are a bunch of things to use as setting lotions instead of the high-priced spreads (commercial ones). If you're in the mood for something completely different, try using:

- *Beer*—preferably opened and left that way for a day or so.
- *The strained water from cooked rice*—cooled off in the fridge, suggested by my friend Louis Gignac, owner of the famous Louis Guy D salon in New York.
- *Skim milk*—applied directly from the carton.
- *Sugar*—dissolved in warm water and combed through.

HOLD-THE-MAYO FRIZZY FIGHTER
(Dry/Normal Hair)

Ingredients:
1 egg
½ cup of mayonnaise

What do you get if you mix an egg with mayonnaise? If you guessed egg salad, you're wrong and if you guessed a super hair conditioner, you're right! Beat the egg and mayonnaise together and spread the mixture onto your hair and scalp. Let it sit for 15 minutes and pray that the man of your dreams doesn't choose that very second to ring your bell. When time's up, shampoo and rinse as usual. Do it once or twice a month to keep your hair frizzy free, and full of bounce.

DIVINE VINEGAR FINISHER

Ingredients:
vinegar
water
2 bowls

How do Mediterranean women maintain their gorgeous hair in their hot dry climates? Well, the secret is vinegar according to

Ahmet, of New York's Coiffeur Ahmet. Wash your hair with baby shampoo and rinse thoroughly. Then mix one part vinegar to five parts lukewarm water. Pour the mixture over your hair and catch the drippings in a bowl. Keep catching, switching bowls, and pouring for about 2 minutes. Rinse well with plain cold water.

LEMON AIDS

In case you haven't heard, lemons are not only wonderful thirst quenchers, but terrific beauty boosters, as well.

LEMON LIGHTEN UP

Shorten the time it takes to lighten up your blond or light brown blah by squeezing one whole lemon over your hair each time you go out into the sun. Massage or comb the lemon juice through to the bitter ends and let the sun shine in.

Bonus: The resulting sun streaks look so natural, only your hairdresser won't know for sure. (He'll think you had an expensive highlighting job behind his back.)

HENNA LEMON AID

Use lemon on your hair too, if you've hennaed it. Lemon helps to maintain henna highlights.

MORE THINGS A LEMON CAN DO FOR YOUR HAIR

Lemons can be used for dark brown and black hair too. Applied before sun exposure, it adds highlights to even the darkest hair.

SQUEAKY CLEAN

Mix lemon juice with warm water and use it as a final shampoo rinse, each time you wash your hair. It cuts through leftover shampoo residue and brings out shine.

MAN THE MANE . . . HAIR CARE FOR MEN

FAKING A GREAT HEAD OF HAIR . . . WHAT TO DO TO MAKE LESS LOOK LIKE MORE

Nothing strikes fear in the hearts of men faster than the thought of losing their hair. The solution is often an abortive attempt to cover the bald spot by combing the remaining hair over it. Unfortunately, when the wind blows, it can look as though the man has a TV antenna growing out of his head.

A more practical solution according to Jack Haber, Editor-in-Chief of *Gentlemen's Quarterly,* is to emphasize what you've got, not what you've lost. If you take a look at some of the magnificant male models in *G.Q.* you'll see some of them haven't any hair up top at all. What have they got that you don't? An understanding hair stylist.

MAN-TENANCE

A man with thinning hair must be especially careful about maintenance too. Daily shampooing, if necessary, is fine because oil-clogged pores, can, in fact, contribute to thinning hair. But put away your blow dryer . . . it can be damaging. You might also consider having a body wave done just at the base to add volume.

QUICK TIPS

Hair stylist Hugh Harrison recommends these quick solutions to make it look as though less is more:

• Use a hair thickener. It will add volume to your hair. So will hair spray. But don't style then spray, do it the other way around. Spray your hair, then brush it through with your head down, brushing from back to front. Then finger-comb into place.

- Raid the women's hair care sections of the store. You'll find the solutions to every sort of hair problem right there.
- Use instant conditioners in place of shampoo every other day or or so. They're quick and easy. Simply apply the conditioner and rinse it out.
- Getting a case of the greys? Use a try-on color which you shampoo in. It will last through about five shampoos.

ILLUSIONS: THE COMB IS QUICKER THAN THE EYE

NOSE-ING AROUND

You may be glad to know that the hair on your head can help to disguise the flaws on your face. For example, if you have a large nose, then you should comb the hair off of your face. Your nose will actually appear smaller. If your nose is too small, then comb your hair onto your face.

FAR-HEADED

Your forehead can be another source of facial imbalance, So, if your high forehead is making you look more like the man from the future than a man with a presence, comb your hair forward or to either side of your face. If your forehead is too low and you look more like a man from the past than a man with a future, you should simply comb your hair forward to cover part of the forehead, or you can comb it back, totally exposing the forehead to make it appear larger. A too wide forehead? Help it by parting your hair high and to the side, which cuts off the temporal area, making it appear narrower.

EAR SHOT

Finally, for ears that can be seen as well as heard, for miles around, have your hair cut, so that it grazes the tops of the ears to cover the heart of the problem.

WHAT'S HOT AND WHAT'S NOT FOR MEN'S HAIR

Hot right now are styles that are ultra short with shorter sides and tapered backs. The curly look is fading, as are Prince Valiant styles. Hair has volume up on the top, but not around the whole head.

AND THEN THERE WERE NONE . . . PERMANENT HAIR REPLACEMENT METHODS

Going bald isn't fun, but for many people, the thought of a hair replacement isn't too many laughs either. Perhaps that's because of all of the confusion associated with hair replacement in general. According to Dr. Peter Linden, New York City plastic surgeon, there are several hair replacement methods available. But just what are they and how much will they cost you? First, and most popular of the permanent methods of hair replacement, is the hair transplant. In a hair transplant, the hair from nonbalding areas is removed and rerooted in the areas of the scalp that are bald.

CANDIDATE DEBATE

Not everyone is a good candidate for a hair transplant. The most likely, successful, transplant candidates? Those with enough hair to cover the balding area. People with coarse, thick, and wavy hair strands are the most likely to succeed. In general, dark hair tends to be coarser than light and has a success rate that is somewhat higher. It is important to realize, too, that when a "plug" (scalp tissue that includes several hair follicles) is removed from the donor areas, it will not grow back there. However, the site is well hidden. A plug of bald scalp tissue is also removed from the bald area where the new plug is placed. There is also a process of waiting, because the follicles fall out before they grow back.

It is, therefore, vitally important that this procedure be done by a qualified physician. He or she is the only person who can medically judge just what your problem is and decide whether the procedure is realistically valid for you. What is the advantage of a transplant over other methods? Once completed, a transplant is your own growing hair and not a temporary replacement. But a transplant may require many sessions to fill in the bald area, and this can be a long haul indeed.

STRIP MINING

Hair stripping is somewhat faster and easier, provided that you have enough thick hair growth elsewhere on the head. In hair stripping, Dr. Linden explained, a whole strip of hair is surgically lifted, left attached by one area of skin, and placed on a corresponding bald area (not unlike the way a peninsula of land is attached to a larger piece of land). That area of scalp is then sewn onto a bald area that is surgically opened. The hair strip is left attached by one section of skin to its original spot to allow for an adequate blood supply to keep the area healthy. Now, what happens to the area that has been "stripped"? The doctor sews that area back up and the sight is hidden by other surrounding hair. Remember the scalp has elasticity, so it will close up without leaving a gaping blank strip.

WEAVING A MAGIC CARPET?

Hair implants, another alternative, involve weaving synthetic hair directly onto the scalp. Dr. Linden does not recommend this procedure for many reasons, most important of which is the fact that whenever a foreign body is attached to *your* body, it can cause serious complications. In fact, many states have outlawed the procedure altogether.

TAKE YOUR HAIR TO DINNER

We hear lots about hair loss and nutrition. According to Louis Gignac, the reality is that most Americans get an adequate supply of vitamins in their diets, and too much of a good thing—including vitamins—can cause the opposite of the sought-for reaction. Poor nutrition, crash dieting, too many goodies, and not enough good food can also cause sudden hair loss.

Other factors that contribute to hair loss are hormonal changes, heredity, age, tension, and certain drugs. Only a doctor can determine which factor, if any, is your fatal flaw.

COLORING BOOK

To be or not to be brunette. Is that your question? Before you end your soliloquy with drastic action, consider these points. Your hair color can dictate your total color statement. Look at the colors you wear most often and think about the ones you'd really like to wear. Will they fit the color you're opting for? Look at your skin color. If you're dark-skinned, ash-blond hair might look bizarre rather than beautiful. If you're very light-skinned, you could look garish rather than gorgeous with black hair.

SWITCH HITTING

Before you make a serious switch from one hair color to another remember that it will be difficult to get your hair color back to its natural shade. Natural hair is made up of several different colors, whereas dyeing gives you one straight color. So you might experiment with try-on colors first. Or try highlighting it if your hair is blond or light brown, or tortoise shelling if it's darker. The other thing to remember is that once you dye your hair, you've got to keep it up. That means coloring it at least once every 4 to 6 weeks, which can be expensive when done professionally and time-consuming, no matter how it's done. But, a wonderful new hair color can do wonders for your ego.

TRY AN EXPERIMENT IN COLOR

Take a true-blue friend with you into a wig or department store. Try on every shade of wig in sight and have your friend snap a Polaroid ™ of you in every different wig. Take the photographs home and put them away for a day or so. Look at them a few days later. Which one makes you feel positively terrific? Which ones aren't so wonderful? Then, go out and do it to it!

FINDING THE RIGHT COLORIST

Whether you want a change of color, or simply a natural looking way to keep your color and just cover the grey, you might consider having it done professionally. If so, how do you find the right person for the job? Here are some tips:

• Word of mouth. If you like the way a friend's hair color looks, find out who does it. That's the best recommendation you can have.
• Don't expect your local barber or beautician necessarily to be as good at coloring hair as he or she is at cutting it. A hair colorist is a professional who only colors hair.
• Don't ask people whose hair is *obviously* colored, about it. If their color is that obvious, it's also obvious that it's not being done correctly.

HOW MUCH?

You'll need to have your hair "touched up" every 4 to 6 weeks. If you opt for a professional touch to your touch up it probably will cost you about $25 and up in major cities. Highlighting or tortoise shelling, which are much more exacting processes, go from $35 to $100 in most metropolitan areas. The actual cost equalizes out, however, because you won't need to have your hair highlighted or tortoise shelled nearly as often as a full coloring.

DO-IT-YOURSELFER TIPS

If you are a do-it-yourselfer, remember that there are several choices available to you. They are:

• *Semipermanent Color*—A shampoo-in type hair color that does not contain peroxide and lasts from four to six shampoos. Good choice if you wish to cover a minimum amount of grey.

• *Henna*—A permanent natural color that is made from plant roots and stems, available in brown, black, and red shades as well as as neutral. Henna (which has been around since the time of the ancient Egyptians) is used to impart color and sheen. Do not use henna if you are more than 15 percent grey, if you've colored your hair, or have recently had a perm. Once it's on your hair, it's usually there to stay. It will change grey to an orangey color which can be attractive if there is minimal greying. If, however, you're out to cover a lot of grey, you may end up with a lot of orange.

• *Rinse*—A temporary color that will last through only one or two shampoos. Effectively covers grey and adds sheen and highlights for a brief period. A rinse will *not* change your hair from dark to light.

• *Permanent Hair Color*—Contains peroxide, and actually changes the natural structure of the hair. Permanent colors can sometimes change the texture of the hair as well, making it coarser and drier.

QUICK COLOR TIPS
Before You Begin

• Coat your hairline (not your hair) from the nape of the neck back up to your forehead with a thick coating of Vaseline® petroleum jelly to prevent the color from staining your skin.

• Do a patch test and leave it on for 24 hours before coloring your hair.

• Check with a colorist if you've had a perm or have straightened your hair recently.
• Don't use a permanent or semipermanent color if you've recently put henna on your hair.

While You're Working

• Always wear rubber gloves.
• If you use a semipermanent foam-in color to cover grey, leave it on about twice as long as the directions indicate.

MAINTAINING THE COLOR YOU DYED TO GET

Does your color-treated hair fade faster than an old soldier? Then here's what Adam Monaco, a colorist with the Gil Ferrar Salon in New York, suggests:

Blond Boom

If your blond comes from a bottle rather than birth, steep a tea bag in 8 ounces of hot water. Pour the cooled liquid into a spray mister and spray through freshly shampooed towel-dried hair. Then comb your wet hair thoroughly and style as usual.

Brunette by Choice

Rather than by chance? Keep the color going strong with a good strong cup of coffee. Not to drink, to pour. Just brew an 8-ounce cup of coffee (regular) and mist your hair with the same technique as mentioned above.

Is Your Red Dead?

Then bring it back to life by mixing 4 ounces of canned beet juice with 4 ounces of water. Again, shampoo, towel-dry your hair, and mist it with the juice.

Rev Up Red, Brighten Up Brown (from colorist Graziella of Resca/Linterman Salon)

Boil a few beets in water. Cool the liquid and pour it over your hair. Or try:

Onion Skin Hair

Boil the skin of one yellow onion, cool the cooking water and pour it through your freshly shampooed hair.

LIGHTEN UP

Want to lighten up your light brown or blond hair very gradually and very naturally? Stan Place, one of the world's renowned beauty experts, came up with this formula: Each time you shampoo, mix one part 20-volume peroxide with one part of your regular shampoo and shampoo as usual. Be sure to mix a fresh batch each time you shampoo, and your hair will begin to lighten very gradually and very naturally.

SILVER THREADS AMONG THE FOLD

One of the most effective ways to cover grey is by combining a semipermanent hair color with henna. The Gil Ferrar Salon does it this natural and extremely safe way:

Apply the semipermanent color to the grey area only, follow with an application of henna over your entire head. Allow the mixture to remain on your hair for about an hour. Shampoo and style. This method of coloring will remove the greyish cast and accentuate natural highlights.

BLACK AND BRONZE
(Puts Bronze Highlights Into Black Hair)

1 ounce of red food coloring
1 ounce of warm water

Mix the food coloring and water together and work it through your hair. Leave it on and dry and style as usual. It is only a temporary, fun way to add highlights and will wash out after your next shampoo.

LEARNING TO FINGER PAINT
(At-Home Highlighting)

Finger painting, you may be pleased to learn, is not just for kids. Finger painting is a great way to put razzle dazzle shine into even the dullest hair. Light up your life-(less) hair with this at-home hair coloring technique, which was introduced by Jean Adams, the Beauty Editor of *Redbook* Magazine.

First buy an all-in-one kit of golden blond one-step permanent cream. After you've read the instructions, brush your hair up, twist it, and pin it back away from your face. Then pull several wispy strands loose at the ears, the nape of the neck, and around your

Finger Painting Is Not Just for Kids. Want highlights without coloring your whole head? Then just "finger paint" random strands around your face.

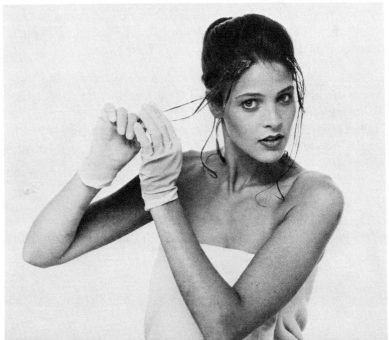

face. Cover your hands with plastic gloves and use your fingertips to "paint" the strands.

Continue in this manner, painting fine random strands at half-inch intervals. Begin at the ears and work toward the top of your head to give the darkest strands around your ears extra time to lighten up. Leave the mixture on your hair for about 10 minutes. Then shampoo and rinse for a sexy, gorgeous head of hair. And as we all know, a sexy, gorgeous head of hair is definitely *NOT* kid stuff!

THE SHAPE OF THINGS TO COME

YOUR HAIR: STYLE IT, WAVE IT, PERM IT, STRAIGHTEN IT

HAIR PLUMPING

Have you ever felt that the only thing that didn't look plump about you was your hair? Well, that's what I call having an ugly day. A good thing to do when you're in the middle of one is to plump your hair. (Or so I tell myself every time I wake up feeling 75 pounds heavier than I did when I fell asleep.) *Here's how:*

- *Dampen It If It's Curly*—Stand in the bathroom and turn on the hot water tap full blast for a few minutes and let the steam go to work for you.
- *Tease It If It's Straight*—Teasing hair is back again, but only if it's done gently with a brush to add fullness . . . not height.

THE GREAT HAIRCUT TEST

To get the cut you deserve, give yourself this test *before* you leave the shop:

After your hair has been cut and dried, shake your head vigorously. Has your hair fallen back into the natural line? Then you've got a great cut . . . if not, get back in the chair and demand a re-cut! After all, you've paid for it and you deserve a fair shear. If it makes you feel embarrassed to be so demanding, think about how embarrassed you'll feel walking into work tomorrow looking like a rooster.

GROWING PAINS

If that wonderful layer cut you got last year won't go away this year, try some of hairdresser Hugh Harrison's favorite tricks.

- Have your hairdresser periodically trim the bottom, to give the other layers a chance to catch up.
- Curl it girl! Nothing disguises what's going on better than a head of curls. Rag ties that you make at home, or even pipe cleaners that you can wrap your hair around, make sensational curls. (Yes, the very ones that your mother tortured your hair with as a child.) Or try using different sized rollers scattered around your head for a change of pace.

Pipe Dreams. Want a head full of tumbling curls? Try pipe cleaners, or even rag strips as curlers. This set is especially good if your hair is growing out.

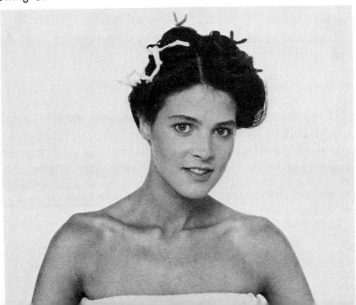

UPTIGHT AND GROWING OUT

Want even tighter curls? Use a setting lotion—either a commercial one, or use one of the for-free ones described in "It's A Natural." For lasting curls while you're having those growing pains, you might consider a perm or body wave.

LIFT IT, NO MATTER WHAT THE SHAPE

Simply drop a comb that has long and short teeth into your hair and lift one section at a time.

THE LONG AND SHORT OF IT

No matter what anyone, including your hairdresser, tells you, long hair on women is sexy. While short hair can be also, long hair is more versatile and lets you look like different women on different days.

BEND WITH THE TRENDS

If you wear your hair chin length or longer, a good basic blunt cut is always in style. Because you can: wave it; straighten it, retro-roll it; French twist it; top knot it; ponytail it; braid it; or leave it (alone).

If you like versatility, don't have your hair cut too short, or in too many layers.

SHORT STUFF

If you like to keep your hair short, and still want to have lots of options with it, try styling it with hair setting gel. It can give you a right-this-second look when you comb your hair into deep waves with plenty of gel and hold it in place with bright combs.

- Pin curl it overnight and wake up to a head of curls.
- Shampoo and finger-dry it for a natural look.

• For all-out glamour, use bright lacquered combs, feathers, or a veiled hat.

MEDIUM COOL

Take a look at any magazine cover. It's like a return to The Sharks and the Jets . . . The Preppies vs. Punks. Which style is right for you? The answer? Whichever one you feel terrific in! Or try a variation on your own theme, by blasting out of your all-American preppie look with a change of pace, à la the *Cosmo* Cover Girl. Or if sexy is your usual style, how about going preppie once in a while?

WHAT'S HOT AND WHAT'S NOT?

What's hot . . . and what's not for hair? Hot are ponytails, French braids, chignons, topknots, and preppie styles. Add dash to preppie hair, with ribbons . . . lots of them worn together as a headband, or wear one alone that matches your eye shadow. What else is hot? If you've got the nerve, try one of the newest bouffant styles. If you don't like it that hot, but want a change, simply change your part. Or slick back one side with combs and gels.

WHAT'S NOT HOT?

Last year's frizzie . . . in fact, it's colder than a fame mane.

GLITTERATI

Want to shimmer and shine? . . . Spray your hair with hairspray, and while it's still wet, sprinkle on some glitter. Spray again. The glitter will stay sprinkled around your hair, giving off bright-light glamour!

NIGHT AND DAY—OFFICE SUPPLIES

Nights are glamorous again, so don't be afraid to go for all-out-drop-dead glamour when it comes to styling your hair for an evening

out. You can even go straight from the office to dinner if you keep
your desk stocked with:

- A brush
- A comb
- A small mister to fluff your hair (if it's curly)
- An assortment of barrettes, silk flowers, and satin ribbons
- Elastic bands to pull your hair back
- Two decorative combs
- Two hair picks (if you've long locks)
- Hair spray
- Extra-long bobby pins
- A curling wand (which has comblike teeth, unlike a plain
  curling iron)

With this assortment of goodies, the difference in your hair will be
like the difference between day and night!

BLOWING IN THE WIND—PRO "CIRCUIT" TRICKS

Did you know that you may not only be drying your wet hair
with your blow dryer, but drying up needed hair and scalp oils as
well? To get the most from your hair dryer, and still leave your hair
in good shape, keep these professional do's and don'ts in mind:

- Don't attempt to dry dripping wet hair. Towel-dry it first to
  get rid of excess moisture. Finger-dry it, then begin to blow dry.
- Do hold your dryer at least 6 inches away from your head
  at all times.
- Do keep the dryer moving. Never concentrate in one spot.
- Do dry the roots first, and ends last, for maximum body.
- Do wrap the just dried hair around a round brush, to keep
  ends curled under. Hold the brush in place until the hair *cools
  completely.*
- Do hold the section of hair being dried downward, for a
  smoother look. For extra lift, angle the section upward.
- Do condition your hair each time you shampoo.

- Don't allow young children to use a dryer unless an adult closely supervises and the lowest heat setting is used.
- Do remember that low airflow is for styling and high airflow is for fast drying.

GET A QUICK CRIMP (LOTS OF TINY WAVES)

To get crimped without getting stuck, simply set your hair when wet, in lots and lots of tiny skinny braids. Secure the bottom of each braid with a colorful rubberband, so that you can even go out with this secret set. When the braids are completely dry, you'll have a full head of crinkly waves!

ENOUGH TO CURL YOUR HAIR—HOME PERMING TIPS

If the thought of giving yourself a home permanent is enough to curl your hair, before you begin, think again. Home perming can give you just the results you want . . . if you know how. But before you take the plunge, take these tips:

- Assemble everything you need before you begin.
- Do a test curl if your hair is color treated or damaged in any way, and don't home perm if you've had henna treatments.
- Start with freshly shampooed hair, so that the lotion can penetrate.
- Don't wind rollers too tightly . . . they should rest comfortably on the scalp.
- If you want tight curls, set your hair. If you want relaxed waves, let the hair dry naturally.

POST PERM TIPS

Don't wash or blow dry your hair for 48 hours after perming, and then let it dry naturally. If you don't wash your hair every day, be sure to mist it each morning before you leave the house. The mist acts as a humidifier to gently tighten the curl.

It's important to use a pH-balanced conditioner each time you shampoo to remove alkaline on newly permed hair. And if you prefer to wash n' wear your hair, don't finger-fluff it until it's completely dry. Too much activity tends to pull the curl out.

Finally, keep a small can of mineral water handy to spray your hair. It's like a ticket to spray . . . and go.

GOING STRAIGHT

If you've always envied straight shiny locks, but couldn't find the key, here's some straight talk from Dr. Jack C. Jaffry, who's been keeping some of the world's most famous heads straight for over 45 years.

The first time that you straighten your hair, have it done by a pro. Only a professional can evaluate the general condition of your hair, the density and the texture, and decide which process is best for you.

HOW TO STRAIGHTEN YOURSELF OUT

There are several methods you might consider if you're thinking about going straight. But remember, all methods straighten existing hair, but *don't* affect new hair growth.

The heat method—if you've ever spent an afternoon with your head dangerously perched on the ironing board, you know that heat straightens hair. You should also know that you can get first- to third-degree burns. DON'T DO IT! EVER!

The chemical method—permanent method in which alkaline swells the hair and alters chemical bonds in the hair itself. Although this is very effective, it must be done carefully.

Reverse waving—not as dangerous, and not as effective.

The newest development, bisulfite, also produces reversible chemical bond changes, and is longer lasting. This method is mainly available through a hairdresser.

2

Your Face is Your Fortune
. . . Cookie!

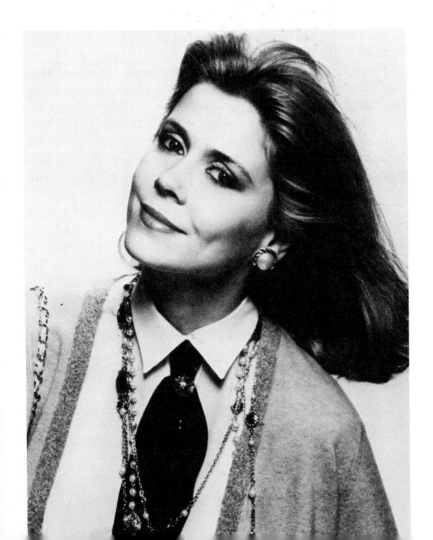

Your face. There it is staring at you every morning in the bathroom mirror. And if you're a female who's managed to make it to age six, chances are good that you have already tried to figure out whether it's round, oval, long, short, oily, dry, and all combinations in between.

Well, we've all done that. In fact, if you were ever asked to conjure up an image of yourself, you'd probably picture your face first. In this chapter you'll find ways to make it up, play it down, clean it, preen it, lift it and learn to love it.

So, let's start with the most visible feature . . . your skin. How much do you know about the skin that you're in? Did you know, for example, that it's the largest organ of your body, and that the thinnest skin of your body is on your eyelids? And if you've ever been troubled with blemishes or acne, it might interest you to know that you're hardly alone. In fact, over 90 percent of all people have acne at one time or another. And that percentage is just as high for many other skin irritations.

So, if you're a determined do-it-yourselfer, or if you'd just like to have some fun with your face, this chapter is for you. But, can making up help you to make it big? Or will gorgeous skin bring you a gorgeous man? Well, I can't promise you that these treatments will cause the masked marvel to swoop down and sweep you off your feet, but I can promise you a few marvelous masques for your face, while you're waiting!

FACE IT

Before you decide to do anything to your face, you should know what type it is.

TRACE YOUR FACE TO FIND YOUR SHAPE

Try this: Pull your hair back. Stand close to a mirror and trace an outline of your face on the mirror—with soap. Voilà! There it is!

SKIN-TYPE TEST

To determine your skin type, wash your face with shaving cream and warm water. Leave your skin alone for 3 hours, so that it regains its natural acidic balance. Then take several pieces of cigarette paper and press them to your cheek, nose, forehead and neck. Where the paper sticks and shows oil spots, your skin is oily. Where the paper doesn't stick, it's dry; and where the paper sticks, but doesn't show oil, your skin is normal.

Skin Flicks. To determine your skin type, you only need a few hours, some shaving cream and cigarette papers.

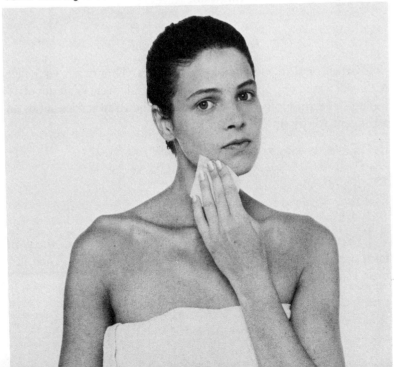

MASKED MARVELS

High-priced facials at top salons are wonderful . . . but not always affordable. If you'd like to find ways to cut corners, and still have beautiful skin, go natural and do it yourself! You can start with ingredients you'll find in your own kitchen. You'll be amazed at how well you wear your food.

OILY SKIN

YOGURT AND YOU
For Drying and Bleaching

Yogurt can have amazing results when you apply it to the outside of your skin. A teaspoon or so of plain yogurt, for example, will help dry up excess oil, and even help bleach scars and dark skin spots. Just apply a bit to your freshly washed face, or scoop some into the palm of your hand and onto your face. Leave it on for 10 minutes and rinse off, for a smoother skin.

STRAWBERRY CRUSH
To Dry Up Excess Oil

Crush or slice some fresh strawberries. Then wash your face with cool water, and spread the strawberries all over. Wait about 10 minutes and rinse off with warm water. The strawberries act as an astringent to dry up excess surface oil.

DR. ZIZMOR'S TOMATO FACIAL
Tightens Pores, Scrubs Skin

1 ripe tomato
3 tablespoons of corn meal

Mash the tomato to a pulp and mix it together with the corn meal. Leave it on for 15 minutes (hide if you want to). Then just rinse your face till it's sparkling clean.

WILD OATS!
Sloughs Off Dead Skin Cells

Oats and other natural grains are marvelous skin sloughers, blackhead removers, and oily skin dryers. Try mixing oatmeal with enough warm water to form a paste. Apply it to your face and let the facial set until it's firm. Loosen the mask by splashing on more warm water. Rinse with a few splashes of cool to completely remove.

OATMEAL SKIN SCRUBS
Cleans While It Sloughs

Low on glow at the end of the day? Then wake your skin up with these super skin scrubs:

1½ teaspoons instant oatmeal (or bran, crushed almonds, or farina)
1½ teaspoons of buttermilk or yogurt

Apply the paste to damp skin and gently massage, concentrating on blackhead areas. The scrub works to help remove dead skin cells and uncover a shiny, healthy underneath.

Extra bonus: Use the same recipe as a mask, by simply allowing the paste to dry on your skin for about 15 minutes, while you lie down with your feet up. Remove the mask with a dry washcloth, and apply a toner if your skin is oily and a moisturizer if it's dry.

MARK TRAYNOR'S SKIN-TIGHTENING BAL MASK

4 egg whites
a bit of lemon juice
a dribble of honey

Mix it up, but don't drink it up. Instead, apply it to the outside of your skin for a skin-tightening mask. Rinse with warm water. After the Bal is over, you'll be fresh enough to dance the night away.

DRY-SKIN MASQUES AND SOOTHERS

DOING THE AVOCADO PEEL

Did you know that hidden inside every avocado is a precious moisturizer? It's right there in the peel. Just peel the avocado and use the inside of the peel to massage your face (or body) gently. Use light upward strokes and then let the oil remain on your face for 15 minutes or so, before splashing it off with three or four handfuls of tepid water.

PETROLEUM JELLY BEAM
For Instant Softness and Glow

Simply warm a tablespoon or so of petroleum jelly over a bowl of hot water and apply the jelly to your freshly washed face. Then bury your face in a towel that's been soaking in warm water, and just relax. Leave the towel on for a few minutes and remove. Wipe the excess petroleum off with a tissue or a cotton ball, and finish up by splashing plenty of warm water onto your face.

BE-WITCH HAZELING
Softens and Moisturizes

Here's a brand new twist on the old favorite you've probably got sitting in your medicine cabinet right now. (It's behind the Band-Aids®.)

2 tablespoons of powdered milk
1 teaspoon of boric acid
Enough witch hazel to form a paste

Mix all of the ingredients together and spread the mixture over your face and neck. Allow it to dry before washing it off with soap and water. Finish up by applying more witch hazel and a good therapeutic type of moisturizer to help seal in the moisture.

The whole treatment costs about 10¢! Now, how's that for a cheap trick?

MASQUES FOR ALL SKIN TYPES

AVOCADO ALTERNATES
To Rev Up Sallow Skin And Close Up Large Pores

Here are two skin soothers for the price of one avocado.

I.

½ avocado mashed
1 tablespoon honey
¼ cup milk

Blend all of the ingredients till smooth at room temperature. Massage the mixture over your face and throat and lie down and relax for 20 minutes. Remove the masque with warm water and a clean cloth or sponge. Top off the facial with a cold water splash or bracing toner.

II.

½ ripe avocado, mashed
½ cup of chilled sour cream

Peel and mash the avocado half and mix it together with the sour cream till smooth. Apply the mixture to your face and lie down with your feet propped up for 20 minutes. Remove with warm water, and follow up with cold to close the pores.

TO SOFTEN SKIN AND BRING UP GLOW

YUMMY HONEY MASQUE

Pull your hair off of your face with a headband. Then apply honey which has been slightly warmed in a saucepan. Test the temperature carefully. It shouldn't be too much above room temperature . . . just warm enough for it to thin out. Spread the mixture over your entire face and leave it on for a full 10 minutes. You can tap your face with your fingers as the masque sits to rev up circulation even more. Rinse the mask off with warm water, and you'll be amazed to see a fresh, go-and-glow skin!

EGG ON YOUR FACIAL

Simply mix together one fresh egg and enough honey to form a paste. Spread the mixture over your face and let it harden into a masque. Then just rinse with warm water to remove. Splash on cold water to soothe.

A FACIAL WITH A SNORKEL
Adds Instant Color, Closes Up Pores

This ice-cold California facial is the hottest thing to hit Movieland since the hot tub. And, my sources tell me that everyone from movie stars to shooting stars are as busy heating their fannies in the hot tub as they are freezing their faces in the kitchen. And as strange as it sounds it really works! (I can vouch only for the faces . . . not the fannies.)

All you need to do is fill a bowl with ice water. Put a snorkel tube in your mouth, and dunk your face to the hairline in the ice water. Breathe through the snorkel tube, and don't search for coral. That's all there is to it. It boosts circulation, and closes the pores temporarily while you have a lot of fun!

APRICOT MASQUE
For A Peaches And Cream Complexion

12 dried apricots
10 seedless grapes
a sprinkle of powdered milk

The California Apricot Advisory Board has developed this fun facial to make at home: Soak 12 dried apricots in water that's already been boiled. Cover and let them sit overnight. Next morning puree the apricots with 10 seedless grapes in your blender. Sprinkle powdered milk to thicken. Spread the mixture over your face and neck and let the facial set for 12 to 15 minutes, then rinse with warm water.

FOR INSTANT RELIEF . . . SPECIAL SHORT-TERM HELPERS

LIFT YOUR SPIRITS AND YOUR FACE
Masque

Ever wanted to look younger or just smoother for a big party? Try this instant years-off masque. It's not a permanent solution, but it *is* a way to make it through the night!

Just separate the whites of 2 eggs and beat them to a froth. Then spread the whites over your clean (very clean) face and throat, making sure to avoid the sensitive eye area. Let the masque dry and rinse with cool water. The egg whites close the pores and tighten the skin, giving you an instant minilift!

GLORIA GAYNOR'S ON-THE-ROAD ASTRINGENT

Disco superstar Gloria Gaynor spends most of her life on the road and needs to be creative about beauty. Let's face it, they don't always have a complete selection of beauty treatments in the outback. When she finds herself on the road and out of astringent she simply rubs an ice cube all over her face, till it feels almost numb. It's an instant astringent . . . and always available.

LIA SCHORR'S SQUEEZE PLAY
Restores pH Balance

This all-natural toner was devised by skin guru, Lia Schorr, and it's even better than most of the commercial ones.

1 lemon
2 ice cubes
$\frac{1}{2}$ teaspoon of wheat germ oil (available in health-food stores)
$\frac{1}{2}$ cup mineral water

Blend all of the ingredients together in a blender, then apply the mixture to your face with a cotton ball. A toner, by the way, is the final step in face cleaning. It restores the pH that can be wiped away with soaps and cleansers.

MASQUES TO SOOTHE SENSITIVE SKIN

TAKE TEA AND SEE
How You Can Miraculously Relieve Irritations and Sunburn

This one's from world-renowned beauty authority, Janet Sartin: Pour 1 cup of boiled water into a bowl. Then steep 2 tea bags in the water and allow to cool to room temperature. Then, using the tea bags as a sponge, gently pat your face. Repeat for a full 5 minutes, dipping the bags back into the solution each time. Blot your skin dry.

Bonus: The cheaper the tea, the better it will be. Cheap teas contain the highest amount of tannic acid and that's what is so soothing to your skin.

MAYONNAISE SUNBURN-SOOTHER

If you've a mild sunburn, simply wash your face with warm water. Then apply the mayonnaise to your face and relax with your feet propped up for 10 minutes. Then rinse gently and rinse again, . . . for quick relief.

MAGIC MILK OF MAGNESIA CLEANSING MASQUE

This one's from *Nine to Five* author, Constance Schrader: If you think of milk of magnesia as something less than the milk of human kindness, you might be surprised to learn that it cleans up the outside as well as it does the inside!

Just spread milk of magnesia generously over your freshly washed face and throat, avoiding the eye area. Let it sit for 15 minutes and remove by spreading another layer of milk of magnesia over the first. Wipe your face and throat gently with a washcloth, soaked in warm water. Rinse thoroughly with tepid water. Follow up by applying slightly warmed olive oil upward with a cotton ball. Leave it on for 5 minutes. Then blot up the excess.

Blemish Bonus: Dab a bit of milk of magnesia on a blemish as soon as you feel it popping up or right after it's shown its ugly head. Apply it to the blemish before bedtime, and by morning it will be on its way to gone.

UNBAGGING YOUR EYES

To get your eyebags unpacked in a jiffy, apply cold . . . any sort of cold, to your eyes and lie down with your feet elevated for one-half hour or so. Particularly soothing are slices of fresh, chilled cucumber, potato, or even wet cold tea bags. There's also a tie-on masque, Aqua-Pac™ by Elsin Products, which is filled with a gel substance and can be chilled in the fridge. The cold shrinks the capillaries which reduces the edema (water retention).

MAKE UP LIKE A PRO

QUICK TIPS AND TRICKS FOR FABULOUS FACES

GOLD FEVER

If you're getting set for a night on the town, and want to look like a million, try gold! All you need is a pot of loose gold-frosted powder and you've got a bronzing kit in a jar. Brush some onto your shoulders and cheekbones. Blend well. After you've applied your regular eye shadow, dab a dot of gold powder onto the center of your top lids as well, and blend. Going bare to there? Then highlight your bosom with a brush of gold, too. If you take care to blend the powder in, you'll get shimmering highlights that pick up the light. But be frugal! You want the look of a golden girl . . . not a golden idol!

CHEEK CHIC

When applying blusher with a brush, begin just under the center of the eye, stroking along the cheek toward the top of the ear. Then apply several thin coats rather than one heavy one. And remember, good brushes are an investment worth making. They last forever with care and can mean the difference between looking good and looking great!

To make your cheekbones appear more prominent, apply a light highlighting cream just above them. Blend well. Then place your blush just below the cheekbones and extend it out toward the temple. You can also apply a brown-tinted contouring powder in the hollow of the cheeks, if you care to.

MAKING LIPSTICK STICK

Dust your lips with powder before applying lipstick, for long-lasting color.

A PERFECT MOUTH WITHOUT A DRAWN-ON LOOK

Outlining your lips with a pencil or lip brush makes a neater looking mouth while preventing the lipstick color from oozing out into tiny lines. If you use a lip pencil, always choose one that is as close to the color of the lipstick as possible. A dark outline with light lipstick looks outdated and artificial.

To create gorgeous lips, use your pencil to make an upside down "V" in the *center* of your upper lip, after you've outlined it. For the bottom lip, draw a line from the ends of your lip to the middle, and draw a few vertical lines from bottom to top. Fill in with lipstick. This technique helps the colors to blend together so that you don't look like you've drawn your mouth onto someone else's lips.

SEXY POUT

For a terrifically sexy mouth, place a dot of gold-frosted powder right smack dab into the center of your bottom lip after you've applied your lipstick. Blend a little, and . . . knock 'em dead!

MAKING UP TO MAKE IT BIG

Making up for the office or school can be tricky. First of all, you probably have fluorescent lighting, which emphasizes everything that might be amiss with skin and makeup. In fact, a face that looks perfectly made up in the gentle light of home can look washed out or overdone in the office. A lighted makeup mirror can help by simulating some of the office conditions. But it also helps to keep a mirror in your desk and check yourself out, in the actual light that you're seen in.

Perfect Mouth Without a Drawn-on Look. Outline your mouth and then go further by drawing a "V" to top and bottom lips, a few vertical lines, and finally filling in with color.

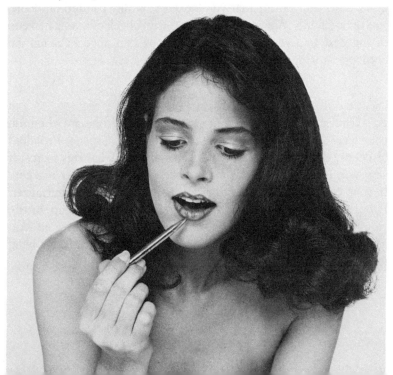

The basic rule for office makeup is to keep it simple. Too much makeup, or makeup that is too obviously applied, can cause you to be taken less seriously than you might like. With eyes, this rule applies: Light emphasizes and dark takes away. If you have large lids, keep them colored with dark shadow (light brown or taupe . . . not black or blue). If you've small, deep-set eyes, on the other hand, bring them out of hiding with a light shadow that extends out toward the temple. Just remember to keep the color natural and the touch light.

MAKEUP SETTER

Once your makeup is fully applied, take an ice cube and gently pat your face with it. The cold plus the moisture sets your makeup for a lovely dewy finish.

MAKING UP PERFECTLY FOR THE BRIGHT LIGHT OF DAY

If you've ever taken great pains to apply your makeup, only to discover to your horror that you looked painfully painted outdoors, you're not alone. We've all done it. Always check out your makeup sitting next to a window to achieve a look that appears as natural outdoors as it does under artificial lighting.

EVEN UP UNEVEN SKIN TONE

Circles under your eyes or an uneven skin tone anywhere on your face? A neutralizer (toner) can help. Amy Greene, President of Beauty Checkers at New York's Henri Bendel, has this secret: If your skin is sallow, use a lavender-based neutralizer under makeup. If your complexion is ruddy or florid, go for a green neutralizer. Dot the neutralizer on with the *tail* end of a makeup brush, around eyes, laugh lines, wherever you need to correct your skin tone. Blend. Apply gently . . . always up and out, before applying foundation.

COLOR CORRECTIONS

Illana Harkavi of Il Makiage suggests that the colors you make up with can make or break any makeup application, no matter how perfect. If you have black skin and hair, start with a red toner, and then choose deep orange and wine tones. Stay away from purple, if you have a greyish cast to your skin, however.

To cover up dark skin spots, use a white toner over spots and under makeup. To conceal broken capillaries, use a lavender toner over the problem spots, before you apply foundation.

QUICK TIPS AND TRICKS FOR FABULOUS FACES

EYELASH DASH

For thicker, longer-looking eyelashes:

• Dust them lightly with baby powder before applying mascara.

• Apply two coats of mascara to both sides of the top and bottom lashes, by applying one coat of mascara to one eye, then moving on to the next. Repeat the procedure on each eye.

• Your mascara will work better and last much longer if you refrain from dipping and dunking the applicator into the container. This causes air to rush in and the mascara to dry out. Instead, pull the applicator out slightly with the wand or brush still inside the container, and rotate the wand for more mascara, more efficiency!

• To keep your eyelashes long, strong, and healthy, be sure to remove mascara each night using a saturated cotton ball . . . not a tissue. Tissues can be abrasive for the delicate skin around the eyes.

• Try baby oil or petroleum jelly, as an eye makeup remover . . . just as good, at half the price.

• Use an eyelash curler before you apply mascara, not after. This will "set" the curl and keep your eyelash curler free of mascara gunk.

• After you've applied mascara, separate the lashes with a special eyelash brush or comb.

BEST BETS FOR BROWS

Want to achieve the look of thick, lush brows, a là Margaux Hemingway or Brooke Shields? Then let your brows grow in, which will take a full 3 months. While they are growing in, use facial bleach on the hairs that you would normally pluck, taking extra care not to get the bleach anywhere near the eyes. This will lighten the new growth temporarily and keep you from looking like an unmade bed while you are going through those growing pains.

• When the brows have grown in, feather them by plucking one or two hairs only out of each section.

Eyelash Dash. For extra thick, extra long lashes, apply mascara to *both* sides of the top *and* bottom lashes.

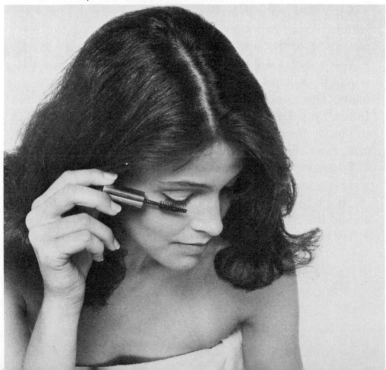

• To get the brow hairs to stay up, moisten a bar of soap and rub an old toothbrush across it, and simply brush up your brows . . . they'll stay that way all day.

• If your brows are very thick, or dark, brush up only the inner edge, the part closest to the nose. It creates the look of thick brows without making you look like you're in shock.

• To achieve a neat, well-cared-for look for brows, begin by first brushing them in reverse with a brow brush or toothbrush. Then smooth them in the natural direction. To darken and accent, add a bit of color to the brush. For a lighter look, dip the brush in loose powder and apply sparingly.

LIGHTEN UP YOUR BROWS

To lighten your brows, beauty authority, Way Bandy, suggests that you use facial bleach. Mix the facial bleach according to the package directions, and apply it to your brows for 2 minutes only. Just be extra careful to avoid the eye area all together. Remove the bleach with a tissue, and wash the area with mild soap and water. Follow up by applying rubbing alcohol to your brows with a cotton ball to remove any residue. The difference is hardly noticeable, especially at first, but the hairs will lighten gradually over the next few hours. Remember, the purpose is to cut the darkness, not to give you blond brows.

COMMON MAKEUP MISTAKES

When it comes to making up, we all make mistakes . . . it's part of the process. And if that weren't enough, we also know that with makeup, like clothing, we've got to keep current to keep chic.

PICTURE PERFECT

Have a friend take a color picture of you. One picture might reveal everything! We all have selective vision, when it comes to looking in the mirror, and we sometimes see what we'd like to see rather than what's actually there.

A SMILE ON THE NILE

Among the more common mistakes is the Cleopatra look (lots of white around eyes which are too heavily rimmed). Aim for more softness, more natural colors.

BLAZING CHEEKS

Suspect that you have blazing cheeks? You may not be blending your blush enough, or maybe it's the wrong color, or maybe it's on the wrong place on your face. Maybe it's all three. To find out what is best for you, try pinching your cheeks. Your blush should be as close to that color as possible. Then smile as you apply your blush, with a dry sponge, so that you can't tell where the color begins and your skin tone ends.

BRIGHT EYES

Bright blue eye shadow dates you. Look for neutrals, such as grey, brown, and smoky shades. They are forever colors.

DOE EYES

Don't. Eyeliner should be softly blended around the eye, not a harsh line that extends beyond the eye itself.

TOO HEAVY AN APPLICATION OF MAKEUP

You just can't conceal bad skin with a heavy application of makeup. You may, in fact, be doing yourself more harm than good by clogging the pores and not allowing your skin to clear and become better. To achieve the most natural skin tone, look for a shade that is closest to your own coloring. And test before you buy. Apply a bit to your neck and blend well. There should be no visible difference between your skin tone and the makeup. If there is, try another shade and another until you meet your match.

OLDER BY ASSOCIATION

If you're still using a look that was popular 10, 15, or even 20 years ago, it's time to hop off that time machine. You may look older simply by looking outdated.

PUTTING IT ALL TOGETHER . . . A MAKEUP ROUTINE YOU CAN LIVE WITH

1. *Cleanse Your Face Thoroughly.* Remove all eye makeup with a special eye makeup remover or petroleum jelly. Then cleanse your face thoroughly with a cleanser formulated for your skin type.

2. *Dot on Toner* (also called neutralizer), wherever skin tone is uneven, with the tail end of an eyeshadow brush. Blend well.

3. *Camouflage Under-Eye Circles* with a moisturizing under-eye cover cream or stick. Although you want to cover dark areas, remember that if it's too light, you will trade dark circles for light rings. So match it as closely as possible to your makeup shade and skin tone.

4. *Apply Foundation.* Remember, always choose foundation by testing it first on the inside of your wrist or on your neck. If you can see a big difference between your skin and the makeup, it's not the right shade for you.

When applying foundation, use a special sponge or your fingers. The latest word from many makeup artists is that nothing smooths makeup on the skin as well as your fingers. Apply one dot of foundation on your forehead, three dots (in a triangle) on your cheeks, and one on your chin. Blend well.

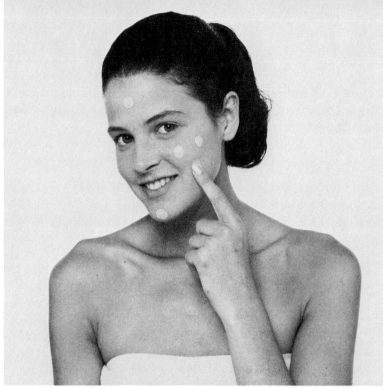

Dot-to-Dot. For a flawless foundation, apply your makeup in this manner before smoothing up and out.

Don't apply foundation to your neck and throat unless you like having ring around the collar.

5. *Set Your Makeup.* A light dusting of translucent powder gently patted over your face will help to "set" the foundation. So will an ice cube.

6. *Make Up Your Eyes.* Color your eyelids with a soft neutral-toned eye pencil, such as a soft brown. Blend well with a shadow brush. Apply a few strokes of a gold-toned pencil in the center of the eyelids for highlight. Blend well. Apply two coats of mascara.

7. *Brush On Blush.* Blusher can be used for contour and color. A brown-toned blush applied in a sideways triangle, with a contour brush, just under the cheekbones and swept back to the ear lobe will create a chiseled look. A rosy tone applied on

the tops of the cheekbones with a blushing brush will make them look more prominent.

8. *Color Your Lips.* Outline your lips as described earlier. Fill in with lipstick that matches lipliner as closely as possible. Finish up with a colorless lip gloss if you care to.

9. *Go Out And Face The World.* You look wonderful!

FIVE-MINUTE MAKEUP ROUTINE

When you need an hour to get ready and don't have five minutes to spare, use this minute makeover: Apply foundation with a cotton swab. Dot it on *only* where your skin tone is *uneven* . . . under your eyes, on your chin or forehead. Then, blend with a dampened sponge. Next, apply a creamy eye shadow, with its own sponge applicator. Place the first smudge of shadow on the outer corners of your lids. Then, go up and outward. Line your lower lids with shadow, using the applicator edge. Blend. Apply *two* coats of mascara to your upper and lower lashes. Dot your cream blush on with your fingertips—along your cheekbones and up toward your temples in an arc—with the *most* color at the *center* of your cheeks. Apply lipstick and you're ready, set, and glowing in minutes.

A BUNCH OF BEAUTY BITS . . . FOR A TINY BIT OF MONEY

Looking for a bunch of beauty bits that won't cost a bundle? Then try some of my favorites:

PENCIL RIGHTING

When your eye pencils get old and brittle, don't toss them out, soak them! Just place the eye pencils point down in a jar of baby lotion and leave them overnight. Wake up the next morning to pencils that will baby your eyes!

DRIED UP BEFORE IT'S USED UP

Mascara or nail polish dried up with lots still left in the bottle? Then place your tightly sealed cosmetics into a bowl of hot water. Use enough water to pretty well cover the products, but not so much that they are floating around. They should stand up in the bowl. The next morning the products will be useable again!

A TRILLION AND ONE USES FOR PETROLEUM JELLY

There's not a whole lot that you can't do a lot with a jar of petroleum jelly and a little ingenuity. For example, use it as a night cream, a makeup remover, a tweezer easer, a chapped skin chaser, and a lip gloss. Petroleum jelly can be used as a perfume primer, too. Just apply some to your pulse spots to make perfume last longer and to keep the fragrance from irritating your skin.

MAGICAL MAKEUP TRICKS

What else can you make with this magic potion? Your own lipstick for starters. Just apply some petroleum jelly to your lips and then smooth a bit of red-tinted eye shadow over that to create a sparkling disco look. Or, next time you get set to get glowing on the town, apply some petroleum jelly to your cheeks, shoulders, and knees. (You can even sprinkle some glitter over that. You'll create your own light show!)

BLUSHING BEAUTY

If you want your blusher to blush far longer, apply some petroleum jelly to your cheeks. Then apply powder blusher right over that. It helps the makeup to adhere without fading. This also works with cream and gel blushers and even with eye shadow.

MONOCHROMATIC COLORS

If you want a coordinated monochromatic look on your face, but don't want to spend the money for matching blusher and lipstick, just buy the lipstick alone. Dot your cheeks with lipstick and cover with a little petroleum jelly. Work both together onto your cheeks. You'll get a high-priced professional look for pennies.

BABY YOURSELF

Another inexpensive way to make up without going broke? Raid the baby products departments. For example, you can use baby lotion as an allover moisturizer, or an under makeup moisturizer. Mix it with your lipstick to color and help soothe chapped lips, at the same time.

Baby powder is another terrific bargain. Use it as a translucent face powder, a dry shampoo, and an under clothing soother. On your kids, it is a great sand remover, on your sheets, it's a summer cooler, and in your shoes . . . well we all know what that's for!

COTTON SWAB SWAP

Swabs make handy inexpensive beauty tools, so swap your swabs and use them to:

• Blend eyeshadow effectively. Swabs are much more hygienic than shadow applicators, which can collect bacteria.
• Swab smudged mascara flecks in a second.
• Remove excess makeup or powder from crevices around your nose, mouth, and eyes.
• Apply acne medication.
• Push back cuticles when manicuring.
• Brush eye shadow onto your eyebrows. It will give them a nice soft color without looking artificial.

RECYCLING PROJECT

Everyone is an impulse buyer when it comes to cosmetics. Well, if you've found that those purchases do nothing more for you than collect dust, recycle them! Try using:

• Moisturizer that didn't sit so well on your face, to smoothe your seat or any other part of your body.
• Cream that disagreed with your face for soaking your hands before a, manicure.
• A facial masque that didn't, on your hands.
• A liquid face cleanser or bath oil as shaving cream for your legs. (It leaves them slick, smooth and, moisturized too.)
• Makeup too thick? Add a drop of astringent (for oily skin) or a drop of freshener (for dry skin) to thin it out.

But remember, discard any product that has separated, discolored, smells bad, causes irritation, or has been sitting around for 2 years or more.

COSMETIC CONSUMER TIPS

• Everyone wants a makeover, so take advantage of a free in-store makeup consultation. But don't feel obliged to buy a product you don't love.
• Experiment at cosmetic counters with pencils, crayons, and sticks before you buy. Remember, you can always erase your mistakes.
• Start by buying the smallest size available of a product you aren't sure of.
• Try colors in combinations . . . the way you'll be wearing them.
• Don't buy a product that you can't try first.
• Always test lip pencils and lipsticks next to each other. How they work together is important.
• Look for hard-textured pencils for the lips and soft-textured pencils for the eyes.
• Try lip colors in all its forms . . . gloss, tint, stick. A color that you might avoid in one form can be more subtle in another.

EYE DO'S . . . FOR EYEGLASSES AND SUNGLASSES

Remember when you would rather have died than wear glasses? Well, glasses are BIG fashion now. After all, what would a preppie be without tortoise shell frames, or a punk rocker without wrap-around "shades"? In fact, it might interest you to know that 75 percent of all glasses sold are nonprescription. And, in fact, the right frames can balance a jutting jaw, thin down a wide forehead or broaden a narrow one.

Here are some tips for choosing the right frames for your face:

• Opposites attract even when you're wearing glasses. So look for a frame that doesn't match the shape of your face.
• If your face is round, look for square or rectangular frames.
• If your face is oval, you can wear any shape—square, rectangular, geometric, or round.
• If you have a square face, look for round or oval frames to soften the contours.
• If you have an oblong face, round or wide oval frames will shorten the look.
• If you have a heart-shaped face, you can be fickle and go for geometric, oval, narrow, rectangular, or square.

CONSUMER EYEGLASS TIPS

• Make sure that the size and shape of the frame fits your face, bridge, and bone structure.
• Temples, or side pieces, must be long enough to fit over your ears comfortably.
• The hinges must be securely implanted in the frame or you may end up with one lens on your forehead and one on your chin. Not chic.

- Glass lenses will be less likely to scratch than plastic, but plastic is half the weight without any difference in optical clarity.
- Even though heavily tinted lenses *look* wonderful, they're murder on your eyes indoors. If you must wear tinted lenses indoors to cut glare from indoor lighting, you should stay with a 10 percent tinted density of grey, brown, or rose.
- Gradiently tinted lenses make eyes look bigger, more dramatic.
- Shades of peach, amber, or brown give a nice glow to cheekbones.
- Sallow skins should stay away from yellowish or greenish casts.
- For maximum sun wear, a dark grey lens is your best choice because it cuts glare the most and distorts vision the least.

EXTENDING EYEGLASS LIFE

So, you've found the perfect glasses: right shape, right color, right price! Here's how you keep them looking as great next year as they do now:

- Plastic lenses should be wet before cleaning and dried with a soft cloth.
- Glass lenses should be cleaned with a nonabrasive cloth.
- Remove glasses with both hands, to keep them aligned. While flicking glasses off with one hand looks great, you'll eventually end up walking with a tilted head to keep your glasses on straight.
- Never place glasses lens-down on a table. Carry a small optical screwdriver with you, so you will be able to tighten loose frames.
- Keep foreign objects, such as pens, pencils, and combs, out of eyeglass cases as a sure way to keep scratches to a minimum.

TOOTH SOOTHE

HOW TO CARE FOR, COMFORT, AND KEEP THOSE PRICELESS PEARLS

TOOTHACHE RELIEVER

To relieve a bad toothache in a flash, try ice. Not on your tooth, on your hand.

Here's how: Turn the hand, on the same side as the toothache, palm up. Place the thumb snugly against the index finger. Notice the bump that forms? That's the "Hoku" point in acupuncture. Now, separate the fingers and massage that point with a piece of ice for 7 minutes. Researchers have found that this treatment will reduce toothache pain in half for 15 to 30 minutes. The procedure can be repeated as often as necessary, or at least until you get to the dentist.

HEADACHE RELIEVER—OR—THE TEETH IN YOUR MOUTH MAY BE CAUSING THE PAIN IN YOUR HEAD

If you've been unable to get any relief from nagging headaches despite tests and time, ask your dentist about TMJ dysfunction which is a lower jaw alignment problem. The condition, according to Dr. Mark Breiner, causes muscle spasms, headaches, dizziness, ringing in the ears and/or an inability to open the mouth wide. If your teeth *are* causing your headaches, a custom-made acrylic appliance for the upper or lower teeth can help the dentist diagnose the condition. If it's found that your lower jaw is improperly aligned and is causing your problem, the bite can be adjusted. This is done by removing small amounts from the teeth in key areas. It may also be necessary for you to have orthodontic work or crowns put in to help finish the alignment and end those headaches once and for all.

SAY NUTS TO CAVITIES

It has recently been discovered that popping peanuts or chunks of cheese after a sweet may help to prevent cavities by steadying the chemical balance in your mouth. The theory is that cheese or peanuts stimulate the flow of saliva, which helps to neutralize the acids that cause tooth decay in the first place. Since these acids thrive on sugar, it would hold that the more saliva, the less acid, and the less acid, the less chance of tooth decay.

So pop a peanut after a sweet (fruit included). But keep it sane, or you may end up with swell teeth and swollen hips.

SEAL A MOLAR

Ask your dentist about sealants for your children's teeth. A sealant is an acrylic glasslike finish which is applied to a child's new permanent teeth before cavities are present or fillings are done. A sealant actually seals off the surface of the tooth, sometimes giving as much as 80 percent decay prevention.

FULL DISCLOSURE

Bacterial plaque—or the monster in your mouth—which causes periodontal disease and tooth decay can be revealed by chewing disclosing tablets. These tablets stain the plaque on your teeth bright red, temporarily. This can give you an idea of where you must concentrate your brushing efforts. (Plaque-free areas will not stain.) Just brush your teeth as usual, then chew on a disclosing tablet. If you're dismayed at the amount of plaque which remains, go on a plaque attack and extend your brushing time by several minutes and increase it to several more times a day.

A WORD TO THE WISE

Don't chew a disclosing tablet right before a night out on the town. The red stain can remain on your teeth for an hour or so making you look like Dracula after a ten corpse meal.

WORTH-A-MINT TIPS

Keep a few sprigs of fresh mint in your desk drawer as a freshener for your breath. When you want a quick breath pick-me-up but don't have the time or the place to brush your teeth, just chew on a piece of fresh mint.

Finally, here's another quick trick: If you run out of toothpaste, always keep in mind that baking soda works as well—and, some dentists say, even better!

BLOODLESS COUP

Having a tooth pulled is bad enough, but when it won't stop bleeding, it becomes sheer misery. If you are ever in this uncomfortable position, take a wet tea bag, fold it in half and bite down. The tannic acid in the tea (which was mentioned earlier as a skin soother) speeds clotting time around the extraction and keeps bleeding to a minimum!

FLOSS FIX

Dental flossing several times a day keeps gums healthy, helps to control plaque, and keeps spaces between teeth free of previously chewed gunk. To use floss properly, wrap a piece around your index fingers, and pull taut. Then simply slide the floss into the spaces between the teeth, and gently up (or down) into the gum tissue that surrounds the base of the teeth. Remove by quickly sliding the floss out, in the opposite direction from which it was inserted.

Bonus Tip: Keep your floss visible so you'll remember to use it! Good places to keep a container are: a desk drawer at work, the shower rack, on your night table.

IF YOU DON'T WANT TO CAP IT, BOND IT!

For teeth that are less than great looking, there is an alternative to capping called "enamel bonding." Enamel bonding is a process in which an enamel-like material is applied directly over a tooth. The material hardens in 20 seconds and probably lasts as long as capping. Enamel bonding is a boon for teeth that are crooked, crowded, widely spaced, discolored, chipped, broken, or even too short. If you've been considering a capping procedure, ask your dentist if you are a candidate for bonding. It costs less than capping and runs approximately $250 per tooth. But take note, enamel bonding, like capping, is not a permanent procedure. Studies show that, when done correctly, bonding lasts about 8 to 10 years. The advantages over capping? The procedure is quick (one office visit). Your teeth won't have to be ground down to nubs, and bonded teeth can be repaired on the spot, should the "enamel" chip or break.

PROBLEMS, PROBLEMS, PROBLEMS . . . AT-HOME TREATMENTS AND MEDICAL SOLUTIONS

DRY SKIN . . . THE FACTS ABOUT YOUR FACE

There seem to be as many misconceptions about dry skin as there are people plagued by it. Here's what's true . . . and what's new about dry skin, according to Dr. Stephen H. Mandy, of Miami, Florida.

First, you should realize that dry skin lacks water, not oil. What you've got to do is replace the water that your skin has lost, so applying moisturizer alone to dry skin *won't* solve your problem. Applying a moisturizer to skin that has already been hydrated (soaked with water) *will* correct it by sealing in the moisture that your skin has already absorbed.

What causes dry skin? Heredity, environment, the forced-hot-air heating and air conditioning in homes and offices, recycled air systems on planes, and water that is too hot, to name a few.

To correct your dry skin problem, begin by cooling off your

bath water . . . and lowering the heat in your home, in the winter. Hot water can actually wash away moisture in your skin, and hot dry air evaporates what moisture is left. In winter, the low humidity outdoors, the dry heat indoors, and the extremes of going from one to the other, can cause your skin, like a concrete road, to crack under the pressure. The same holds true if you spend much of the summer sealed up in an air-conditioned office or home.

What to do? Spritz your face with mineral water throughout the day, *then* use a good therapeutic moisturizer, before you make up each morning if you're a woman, and after shaving if you're a man. Do the same to your damp face each evening before you bed down.

And if you think that you should use a moisturizing makeup and forget about the rest, think again. A foundation is for cover-up and not for moisturizing, per se. Most foundations contain talc or a similar substance and can actually pull water away from the skin. A good moisturizer can seal in the water by coating the skin. This "coating" will also set up a barrier between the environment and your skin.

GOOD MOISTURIZERS

Try: Lacticare™ from Stiefel Laboratories, Keri™ Lotion from Westwood Pharmaceuticals, and Creme Santal Face Treatment Cream™ from Clarins, Paris.

REMEMBER, great skin, unlike royal blood, is not something you have to be born with, but it *is* something you can create!

WHAT'S THE DIFFERENCE BETWEEN DRY SKIN AND WRINKLES?

Dry-skin lines and cracks are not wrinkles. Dry-skin lines (those hairline cracks that can appear around your nose, forehead and mouth) are surface skin problems caused by the conditions just described and can be corrected.

Wrinkles, however, are the result of a loss of elasticity *beneath* the skin surface, when the collagen fibers and elastic tissue break down. Moisturizers simply cannot correct and rejuvenate tissue *below* the skin surface.

Wrinkles are, however, an eventual fact of life for everyone. It's just a matter of how early or how late you develop them. Wrinkles that don't go away will make their debut in your life based on sun exposure, heredity; sun exposure, stress; sun exposure, the amount of melanin in your skin; and, sun exposure. So, if you can't change your family, the amount of stress you're under, or the amount of melanin in your skin, at least change the way you sit (or better, *don't* sit) in the sun.

SCREENING YOURSELF

Theoretically, we should apply a sunscreen to all exposed skin every day of our lives to prevent . . . or at least . . . delay the onset of wrinkles. (That includes hands, face, and neck.) An application of sunscreen, under your makeup if you're a woman or after shaving if you're a man, takes 2 minutes and will help keep the sun from shining in and prematurely aging your skin. Remember, the sun shines all year long so you should use sunscreen all year long. Be especially careful to apply sunscreen before you hit the ski slopes because snow, like sand, acts as a giant sun reflector to magnify the intensity of the sun's rays. And always cover the most delicate part of your body—the skin around the eyes—with sunglasses.

ACNE . . . MYTHS, METHODS, PROBLEMS, SOLUTIONS

Did you know that the term "acne" is not only reserved for severe scarring conditions, but for the once-a-year pimple as well? People throughout the ages have conjured up myths about why skin breaks out. Even medical experts do not agree. In controlled experiments, researchers have found that diet seems to have little effect on acne. But most doctors still maintain that if you find that certain foods do cause *you* to have skin problems, you should stay away from them. And it's also good to remember that while chocolate, fried foods, and other previously banned goodies may rarely cause you to break out in acne, they *will* cause you to break out in large hips . . . always.

And what about sex? Remember hearing that a good roll in the back seat of a Chevy was guaranteed to clear up your complexion? Sorry, but there's not a back seat, brass bed, or beach boy in existence that can help you to clear up your skin. Sex just has nothing whatever to do with acne. (Unless anxiety over sex or the lack of it causes you to worry and therefore break out in pimples.) The myth was probably born of the fact that skin erupts when hormones are in flux, as they are during puberty or the teen years. And androgen, a male sex hormone (which is found in both men and women), can be the reason by causing an enlargement of oil glands, and the oversecretion of oil. When excess oil is secreted, the oil gland may enlarge its opening, plug up, and produce a pimple (technically known as an acne lesion). Skin bacteria also seems to play a role in the process, as do the hair follicles.

The most important factor is probably heredity. And since you can't change your family, you can change your skin care routine. *Here's how:*

ACNE DO'S AND DON'TS

• Don't pick or squeeze blemishes; they can open, spreading infection.
• Don't experiment with your friend's cosmetics. That's a good way to spread germs.
• Don't use a moisturizer. A moisturizer is great for dry skin, but not for oily.
• Don't eat foods that you know will cause you to break out.

Different foods cause different reactions in different people. So stay away from the ones that cause you trouble.

• Don't be afraid to get professional help when you need it. Untreated, acne can cause you unnecessary scarring, pitted skin, and unhappiness.

• Do change your bed linens and towels frequently. Keep your hands . . . and your hair . . . away from your face. Excess oil and dandruff can fall from your hair and onto your face, so it's important to use a shampoo for oily hair or dandruff and to use it frequently.

• Do use a stronger cleanser 2 weeks before menstruation, to combat your overactive oil glands if you are a young woman.

• Do get plenty of rest and fresh air and eat a well-balanced diet.

• Don't use heavy, oil-based cosmetics. They can clog pores, making your skin worse.

• Don't be fooled by the term "Hypo-Allergenic." Those makeups are designed for allergies—not acne.

IT'S A WASHOUT

Are you a washout at washing up? Dr. Jonathan Zizmor, author and dermatologist, developed this wash routine, for super cleaning:

• Soak a terry washcloth in a sink filled with lukewarm water and wet your entire face and neck.

• Work up a rich lather and gently scrub your face with the cloth.

• Relather the cloth and place your fingertips inside and scrub around each blemish in a circular motion for 2 minutes.

• Rinse the cloth, refill the sink, and use the cloth to remove the lather.

• Cup your hands and splash your face with water until the soap residue is gone.

• Pat dry and apply acne medication.

DAILY REGIMEN FOR ACNE

Dr. Kenneth Flandemeyer, author of the book *Clear Skin,* recommends that you wash your skin several times a day, and apply a drying and peeling agent (such as a benzoyl peroxide lotion) each and every time you wash. Acne is an aggressive skin condition, so to fight it, *you* must be aggressive.

• Begin with 5 percent benzoyl peroxide, and gradually work up to 10 percent. Since these medications are strong, you may be dismayed at the first skin reactions that you get (red, dry patched), but the medication *does* do the job and your acne will not only begin to clear up, but you'll see that a regular regimen works as a preventive to future breakouts.

• When you find a routine that works for you, stick with it. Remember, there is *no* cure for acne . . . only help. But to *keep* clear, you've got to keep your routine up, even after you *have* cleared up.

• Summer sun brings its own benefits, so you can keep your skin care routine lighter, when you spend time outdoors. But that doesn't mean that you should bake in the sun! Minimal amounts of sun will help to dry and peel your skin, too much will ruin it.

THE SERIOUS SIDE OF ACNE

What if your condition is more serious? What can a dermatologist do for you? New York's Dr. Hillard Pearlstein says that simple drying and peeling lotions used under strict supervision may be enough. If not, locally applied topical or internal antibiotics may be needed. In severe cases, hormonal therapy, such as cortisone derivatives, may even be necessary. Surgical drainage of the lesions by the doctor may be recommended for the most severe cases.

WHEN SHOULD YOU SEE A DOCTOR?

When you feel that you can't handle your skin problem alone; and if you have more than a few pimples, or if any pimple takes on a cystlike quality.

Acne is too often a condition that leaves the victim with severely scarred skin, which is completely unnecessary. And, only a doctor can keep a potential worry from becoming a real-life disaster.

DR. ZIZMOR'S AMAZING ACNE ASTRINGENT

½ cup of witch hazel
½ cup of rubbing alcohol
a pinch of alum
a pinch of mint extract

Mix all ingredients together and apply the astringent to your face at 10 A.M., 2 P.M., and 4 P.M. It really works wonders!

DR. ZIZMOR'S AMAZING ACNE MASK

2 teaspoons of any acne cream or lotion
2 teaspoons of Fuller's earth (available from your druggist)

Mix the ingredients into a paste, apply evenly to your face, and leave on for 20 minutes.

Rinse it off with cool water, for tighter, smoother skin.

A Note Worth Noting: Remember, there is *no* cure for acne. Any of these treatments, used alone or in combination, will help to dry up and clear up your skin temporarily. But, if you are already under a doctor's care, be sure to check with him before you do anything to your skin.

CORRECTIVE COSMETIC SURGERY

What can cosmetic surgery do to correct what age, stress, or heredity have done, not only to your face, but to other areas of your body as well? For the answers we went to a New York plastic surgeon, Doctor Peter J. Linden.

The most important consideration is *why* you want to have surgery to change a part of you in the first place. You should be able to point out specifically the cause of your distress or discomfort, and you should be able to discuss your expectations in detail with your doctor. Corrective surgery can give you an incredible added sense of self-confidence, but it is not a panacea for your life!

WHERE, WHAT, AND HOW?

Plastic surgery, which used to be thought of as the hidden resource of the rich and famous, is now something that people from all walks of life are turning to as a means of altering, enhancing, or even rejuvenating the appearance of parts of their bodies that have made them uncomfortable, or even miserable. What is possible with corrective surgery? And, what isn't? Let's start with the nose.

A NOSE IS A NOSE?

Nasal plastic surgery is still one of the top operations requested, both for adults and mature teens. If you've been contemplating this procedure, look critically at your face in a three-way mirror.

Your critical self-evaluation is crucial in working with your plastic surgeon. You both must have the same goal in mind for you to feel happy with the results. You must also be willing to listen to your doctor and know beforehand what the limitations of your particular surgery will be.

The actual surgery is performed inside the nose so there are no external scars at all unless nostril reshaping is needed.

TAKING IT ON THE CHIN

If you've decided that one chin is better than none and infinitely better than two, you might be interested to know that chin surgery is one of the simplest and most dramatic of all procedures. To correct a receding chin, the surgeon simply inserts a tiny silicone-filled, airtight implant (a sac, which feels like human tissue with silicone trapped inside the sac). The implant will very quickly become surrounded by scar tissue which holds the implant in place forever. Voilà! Your face is brought into proportion and the receding chin is brought out and into balance with the rest of your face.

For sagging jawlines or to remove the "turkey gobbler" skin and fat from the neck and chin, a full facelift must be performed to prevent folds or "pleats." Having the neck and chin done without doing the face would be, in effect, like altering a sleeve by pulling and tucking the fabric in the center of the arm, instead of at the cuff or shoulder.

ERASING LINES, WRINKLES, AND ACNE SCARS
The Collagen Connection

By now, you've heard lots about collagen creams, lotions, and potions. Well, according to several sources, the molecules in collagen are larger than the cell structure of human skin, so applying a collagen cream won't help too much. It just can't be absorbed properly. Dr. Linden explained that the newest treatment for lines, wrinkles, and pitted or pockmarked skin involves collagen injections. Collagen, a natural protein, is injected into the skin depressions, plumping them out to align with the surface of the healthy skin around it. This process builds the skin up, rather than planing it down, as is done in chemical peeling and dermabrasion.

Since collagen is a naturally occurring protein found in skin, the skin accepts the substance as its own. Your doctor would have to give you a test dose 1 month prior to treatment to test for possible adverse reactions.

What About Silicone?

Silicone, unlike collagen, is a synthetic material. And any synthetic material that is injected into the skin can have serious and dreadful side effects. While the synthetic substance does plump out the skin in much the same way that collagen does, silicone is still an artificial foreign body. The results have sometimes been so disastrous that this procedure has been banned in many states. The problems include thick scar tissue formation around the injection site causing lumps, bumps, and permanent discoloration or bright red splotching of the skin. Most silicone problems can *not* be repaired.

THE EYES HAVE IT

If you think you'd like to get your eyes "done" take this simple test: Stand in front of a mirror and look to see if the skin of the upper lid extends almost to, or beyond, the eyelash line. You don't need a test for the lower lid, you already know if it's necessary.

Plastic surgery of the upper lid will get rid of the hoods of skin and fat that can cause you to look older and even hamper your vision. Lower lid surgery removes the heavy fat pockets and some of the wrinkled skin to correct a tired, dissipated look.

The operation is very quick and the results can take years off your appearance.

DERMABRASION AND CHEMICAL PEELING

With both procedures some of the outer skin layers are planed down so that the lines, wrinkles, or scars are reduced. With dermabrasion this is accomplished with a burr. With chemical peeling, the procedure is performed with masks. There are drawbacks, however, such as possible depigmentation blotches that won't disappear. You should be especially careful if you are light-skinned, or a natural blond or redhead.

LITTLE THINGS MEAN A LOT

Little things mean a lot, especially when those little things have come to reside on your face. Small broken capillaries, for example, aren't earth shattering, but they are annoying. They can be caused by many things—such as cold weather, hot water, even alcohol. But they can be easily treated in a doctor's office with a very mild cautery treatment. A tiny needle injected at the site completely obliterates the unsightly capillaries on the spot in one office visit.

SHAVING YOUR LIP

Many people, men as well as women, are having their lips surgically shaved to remove fine lines, wrinkles, and puckering. The new procedure, when done by a qualified surgeon, is fast, reliable, and easy. If your lipstick "bleeds" or if your mouth looks as if it's puckered up, even when it's not, your doctor can simply "shave" the outer skin layers. This will expose the healthy unlined skin underneath. The results? A dramatic difference which will make you look younger and neater.

ARE YOU A CANDIDATE?

Not everyone is a good candidate for plastic surgery. In fact, since cosmetic surgery has grown so popular in the last few years, many people have been consulting with doctors only to be told that surgery isn't for them. And plastic surgery isn't for you if:

- You're in poor health or have certain chronic diseases.
- You see plastic surgery as an out for an emotional problem.
- You're planning to lose weight. Your body structure changes with weight loss, so lose the weight first.
- You want to have surgery to please someone else. If you choose to have elective surgery it should be for *you*. Not your lover. Not your spouse. Not your parents. Just you.

IS YOUR SURGEON A CANDIDATE?

Before you choose a plastic surgeon, check his or her credentials. Is your surgeon board-certified in plastic surgery? Board certification in this speciality is extremely difficult to achieve and only the most highly qualified surgeons make it. Make sure, too, that the certification is in plastic surgery and not in another specialty.

• Ask to see pictures of previous patients and don't be intimidated. After all, it's your face.
• Ask your friends who've had cosmetic surgery what they thought of their results. If you can tell that someone has had a "nose job," for example, it isn't a good one.
• Stay away from surgeons who have a noticeable "style." You don't want the stamp of a particular surgeon on your nose. You want a surgeon who is interested in doing what's right for you, not one who stamps out assembly-line faces.
• Most important, be sure your surgeon has been selected on the basis of mutual trust and respect.

LIFE AFTER LIFT . . . THE POSTOPERATIVE PERIOD

Most operations are done under local anesthetic and last between 2 to 4 hours. Patients usually experience discomfort, not pain, and recovery is remarkably quick. Even for a full facelift you can be back at work in a week or two. With a good plastic surgeon, scarring is minimal. It's normally hidden inside the nose for a rhinoplasty, in a natural flesh crease such as the eye area or the hairline for a facelift.

3
Body Shop . . .

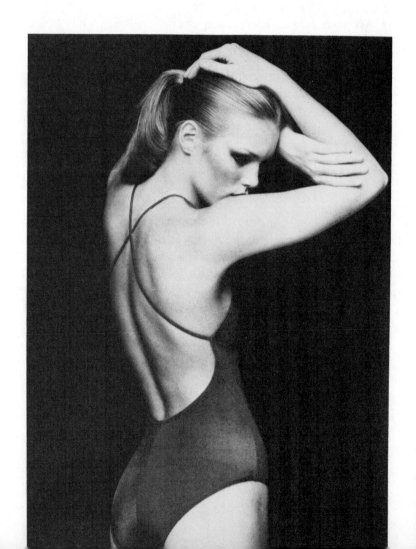

Do you know how to speak body language? You do if you can get your body to look the way you say you want it to, but you don't if you talk a good game, hope for the best, and it never happens.

In this chapter, we'll tell you the secret tricks of the trade . . . the ones that the pros use to slim down, shape up, build up, and tone it all. We'll also give you tests to judge the shape you take, and the very possible shape of things to come.

TESTS, TIPS, TRIED AND TRUES TO ACCURATELY EVALUATE WHAT SHAPE YOUR SHAPE IS IN

To get the answer to the ultimate question, you needn't rely on scales and height/weight charts alone. Here are some other tests which may be even more effective ways of answering the big question.

- *Mirror, Mirror on the Wall.* Unless you live in a fun house, it won't lie. What you see is what you've got. At least once a week, strip down in front of a full-length mirror and have a long, hard look. Then turn around and hold a hand mirror over your shoulder to get a good insight into your hindsight.
- *The Yardstick Test.* Lie flat on your back, place the middle of a yardstick—lengthwise—on your stomach. If your stomach keeps the ends from touching both your chest and your pubic bone, you probably are above your ideal weight.
- *The Tape Test.* Take a tape measure and measure your bustline, thigh, calf, and ankle. You are probably overweight

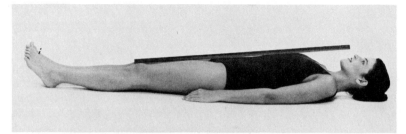

Am I Really Too Fat? For a sure fire answer, try the yardstick test. (You can also use a plain stick for this one.)

if: Your bustline is more than 9 inches larger than your waistline, your hips are more than 3 inches larger than your bust, your thigh is more than 8 inches larger than your calf, or if your calf is more than 6 inches larger than your ankle. Finally, measure your neck and calf. If your neck is the same as, or larger than, your calf, you'd better not wait for the cows to come home to start dieting.

PINCH AN INCH

If you suspect that you're on the road to fat city or have already reached that unhappy destination, try this test to tell for sure:

Pinch the skin directly under the navel between your thumb and forefinger. Generally, a man who is within his right weight range will not be able to pinch more than 1 inch of skin. A woman should not be able to pinch more than 1½ inches of flesh. If you've failed, you can either lose weight or move to the Via Venetto where having lots of flesh to pinch is wonderful!

FINDING YOUR FRAME

"Ideal weight charts" are tricky little devils. And no one can ever decide whether they're large-, medium-, or small-framed. Well, if you're like most of us, you probably look under the large frame whenever you've managed to consume a box of chocolate chip cookies. If the confusion has bothered you, however, here's the ultimate answer. And once you've measured yourself, you can never be fooled again. Sorry.

Take a tape measure and measure your wrist. A small-framed woman will have a wrist measurement of about 5½ inches, a medium-framed woman will have a wrist measurement of about 6 inches, and a large-framed woman will measure in at about 6½ inches.

OTHER WEIGHT CHARTINGS

Remember, too, that weight charts are usually calculated for women wearing 2-inch heels and who are 25 and older. So always add 2 inches to your height. And if you are between 18 and 25, subtract 1 pound for each year under 25 to chart your correct weight.

DO IT OR DIET

In this section we'll give you a load of tricks and tips for dieting. We want to give you the incentives and the strategies that can help keep you on your course. We won't outline a specific diet, only a doctor or a licensed weight-loss group can do that for you in person. But remember, *crash diets don't work and are dangerous*. In fact, recent evidence proves that the longer it takes you to lose weight, the longer the weight is likely to stay off. And every bit of evidence points to the fact that fad diets are just that. To lose weight permanently, you've got to do it sensibly, with a well-balanced diet of good nutritious food.

And remember, before you start any weight-loss program, see your doctor.

If you've been on a diet since birth and all you've ever lost is your mind, you may well have the will, but not the power to stick to a diet. You may also not have all of the facts. Herewith, the facts:

INCENTIVES, TIPS, AND LITTLE-KNOWN WORKABLE SOLUTIONS

CALORIE CLUES

Thirty-five hundred calories equal 1 pound of fat. You will gain a pound if you take in 3,500 more calories than your body needs, to maintain a certain weight, and you will lose a pound if you take in 3,500 less than you need.

DIETING TIPS AND TRICKS

• Alcohol and fat are the most concentrated foods, and alcohol is the only food that is directly absorbed by the stomach. In fact, the body uses alcohol before it uses fat as fuel. Cut down on both.

• Drink five glasses of fluids a day when you aren't dieting and seven to eight glasses when you are. An 8-ounce glass of water before meals will also act as a buffer for hunger pangs. *Remember:* Many diet soft drinks, though low in calories, do contain fluid-retaining sodium. So do many frozen and canned foods.

• Exercise more. Exercise not only burns calories, but also reduces your appetite.

• Think about your 20-minute belly button. It takes 20 minutes for the brain to get the message from the stomach that it's full. You can consume a mountain of unneeded calories in 20 minutes, and that's what accounts for that stuffed feeling you're often hit with when it's too late. Wait 20 minutes before you have dessert, and you may find that you won't feel like having any dessert at all.

• Be kind to yourself. If you do slip off the diet wagon and onto the ice cream cart, don't use this as an excuse to quit. A slip of the lip doesn't mean lifelong failure. Get back to your diet immediately, if not sooner.

• If you know a stressful situation is coming up, eat a nutritious meal beforehand. You'll feel calmer and stronger for the effort. Too often, stress leads to hunger.

• Leave a small amount of food on your plate . . . ALWAYS . . . as an exercise in self-control.

• Avoid sugar and junk foods. Actually, nutritious foods (while not as much fun) do satisfy your body's needs and fill you up. Sweets just don't.

• Put away your salt shaker. Your body needs only $1\frac{1}{2}$ to 2 grams of salt per day. You get more than that much from natural salts in food.

• Don't sample and taste foods during preparation. You can unintentionally devour a whole meal in little samples.

• Make a formal sitting of it EVERY TIME you eat. Have you ever noticed how standing up nibbling from the fridge somehow doesn't seem to count? It does.

• Keep a food diary. In it write down every morsel that you consume . . . you may be shocked at how much you munch that you are unaware of.

CALORIE CUTTERS

Try steaming, poaching, and broiling as many foods as possible. When broiling or baking, use lemon juice or bouillon to moisten the pan, instead of butter or fat.

Trim the skin and fat from meat or poultry before cooking.

HOW YOU EAT IS IMPORTANT, TOO

Adele Davis was right when she said that you should eat breakfast like a king, lunch like a prince, and dinner like a pauper. Breakfast is your most important meal. It supplies energy for the day, and gets your metabolism moving.

INCENTIVES

If there's no doubt about the fact that you'll be occupying more space this year than last, stop hitting yourself over the head and try giving yourself incentives, instead. For example:

- Put on your your skimpiest bathing suit and stand in front of a full-length mirror. Then turn around and hold a pocket mirror over your shoulder to get some insight into your hindsight.
- Tack a thin picture of yourself or someone else on the refrigerator and cupboard doors. It helps to remind you of why you don't want to eat.
- Aim toward a goal such as a dazzling new bathing suit, or strapless evening dress.
- If you can't help but splurge on junk food, then do so as you look into a mirror. And watch yourself as you take every bite.
- Join a group such as Weight Watchers. Not only are they inspirational, they're encouraging.

GREAT EXPECTATIONS

Successful dieting is sort of like the story of the tortoise and the hare: Slow and steady wins the race. So, if you've ever started dieting and expected to miraculously wake up thin 2 weeks later, you've been a victim of great expectations. Remember, you didn't become overweight overnight, and you won't become thin overnight!

PROPER EXPECTATIONS

With a sound weight-loss program, you can expect to lose between 1 to 2 pounds a week. You may, in fact, lose more than that at the very start and lose less than that as you progress. And remember, you won't lose faster if you skip meals. In fact, it might actually slow you down.

THE LAST PLATEAU . . . OR WHY YOU'VE STOPPED DROPPING WEIGHT EVEN THOUGH YOU SEEM TO BE DOING EVERYTHING RIGHT

Even if you do diet sensibly, you may reach a discouraging stage called a plateau. This is the time when you can't seem to drop another ounce, and it's also the time when many dieters get discouraged and give up. DON'T! There are many reasons for interrupted weight loss. They are:

• Tissue and skin may not shrink as quickly as the fat that is being lost, particularly as you approach middle age. The excess space can hold fluids. But the fluids will pass as the skin and tissue shrink back.
• A severe sunburn, a sudden increase in exercise, or even a fever can cause your body to retain fluids. So reduce your salt and caffeine intake during these times.
• There is a theory, too, that your body has a memory of a time in your life when you held a certain weight for 5 years or more. You may find yourself temporarily plateaued back there again. Most importantly, don't get discouraged. This too shall pass.

FOOD FOR THOUGHT

• Think not only about what you eat, but what you add. For example, mayonnaise adds 85 more calories per sandwich than mustard, and every tablespoon of ketchup contains about 1 teaspoon of sugar!
• Potato chips have 45 calories more per cup than popcorn. An oatmeal cookie is 33 calories more than a graham cracker. A slice of pizza weighs in at about 200 calories, while a burger with cheese is more like 500!
• If a recipe calls for bacon, use small amounts of smoked yeast instead. Substitute corn oil for butter, arrowroot flour for regular flour. And just eliminate MSG all together. If your recipe

calls for black or white pepper, use cayenne instead and for salt, substitute minced fresh garlic, minced celery, shallots, tangy spices, even dried herbs.

So train yourself to *think* before you add, eat, or binge.

WHEN NOT TO EAT

Nibbling is a form of bingeing so:

• Don't nibble when you're on the telephone . . . it's not only an unconscious way to eat without thinking, it's also a great way to annoy whomever you're speaking with.
• Don't nibble or eat anything in front of the TV set. It's a killer.
• Don't eat while reading or driving, they require too much concentration on the act and too little on the eat.

Other stimuli for bingeing . . . of any sort . . . are loneliness, or worse, just being alone. We've learned, you see, not to pig out in front of others but still have a little problem doing it alone. Just remember, that bingeing in private isn't your personal secret, it becomes quite public whenever you must face a bathing suit, and a beach. Besides, we know that bingeing makes us unhappy and unhappiness makes us lonely, and so on and on.

Try to discover what prompts *you* to munch. The discovery shouldn't surprise you. After all, all programming is a form of learning, and, overeating is learned behavior.

EXORCISE IT . . . WITH EXERCISE

You *know* that diet alone doesn't do it, so now's the time to tone it, while you trim it. Here are a bunch of ways to do just that, while learning facts that will astound, amaze, and encourage.

PRO EXERCISES TO SHAPE UP AND TRIM DOWN

THE ENDURANCE TEST

If you are under 25, but feeling over the hill physically, take the quick endurance test to determine how fit . . . or unfit . . . you really are:

Stand with your feet, shoulder width apart, and your toes pointing forward. Then squat down till your knee joints form a 90° angle. If you can manage 75 or more knee squats, you're practically an Olympic contender (if there were an Olympic squatting squad). If you can manage 30 or more, you're still in good shape. Fifteen or less? Then think about taking up an exercise regimen . . . soon!

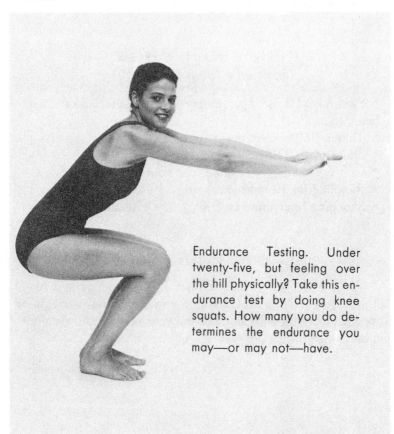

Endurance Testing. Under twenty-five, but feeling over the hill physically? Take this endurance test by doing knee squats. How many you do determines the endurance you may—or may not—have.

HOW MUCH AND HOW MANY

Have you ever wondered how long it would take you to exercise away an apple or sleep off a hamburger? The Campbell Soup Company has published a very interesting little paperback called "Your Active Way to Weight Control" which is part of their "Turn-Around Program." Here are some of the facts:

The less you weigh, the longer it will take you to burn off calories. And every activity, from watching TV to cleaning the house to even eating, burns calories. In fact, eating burns between 80 to 95, per hour, depending on your weight. Now, back to that apple. If you now weigh 120 pounds, it will take you 41 minutes of housework, or 69 minutes of watching TV, or 8 minutes of running to burn off just one 75-calorie apple. And if you can bear it, it will take you four times as long to burn off your burger.

ENERGY-EFFICIENT EXERCISES
(Based on a 120 pound person)

- Swimming (45 yards per minute) burns over 600 calories per hour
- Tennis: 380 calories per hour
- Office work: 130 calories per hour
- Coffee klatching: 85 calories per hour
- Bicycling (at 10 miles per hour): 310 calories per hour
- Shopping (everyone's favorite sport): 150 calories per hour

WALK AWAY TEN POUNDS

Want to be 10 pounds thinner 1 year from now, without dieting? Then walk. A brisk 20-minute walk each day will trim off 10 pounds in 1 year without changing your normal eating patterns one bit.

BURN CALORIES WHILE SITTING

Are you a mover? Well, if you're one of those people whose mother always complained that you could never sit still, you're probably thinner than the kids who could because moving around burns calories. Slim people are generally on the move, while heavy people are static. Slim people shift in their chairs, cross and uncross their legs, talk with their hands, wiggle from side to side.

The active sitter may actually burn up 25 calories more per hour than the inactive sitter. Since we sit on the average of 15 hours a day, it adds up to 136,000 calories a year which adds up to a whopping 39 pounds!

So, if you're a sedentary sitter, get a move on. Start shifting around, cross and uncross those legs, use your hands to gesture, use the stairs instead of the elevator, park your car at the farthest point in the parking lot; take the dog for an extra walk! After all, the calories you burn will be your own!

LEGS, LEGS, LEGS

WHAT TO DO FOR THEM

LOCKED UP IN CELLULITE

Have you ever asked yourself: What is cellulite and why has it chosen my thighs to live on? If you have, you're not alone. Cellulite has been defined as a gel-like substance made up of fat, water, and wastes in immovable pockets just beneath the skin. But many doctors believe that cellulite is no different from ordinary fat and actually doesn't exist at all.

Well, if you believe that it does exist and it exists on *your* body, take this test to find out for sure: Squeeze the flesh between the thumb and index finger. If it ripples and looks more like an orange than a thigh (or a bottom of a stomach), you've got it . . . even if there is no such thing.

UNLOCKING IT

Every expert questioned on the subject agrees that good nutrition or, more precisely, the lack of it, is the major culprit in causing cellulite and is the key to unlocking it.

So, be sure to:

• Drink 6 to 8 glasses of water per day (or more) to flush your system of fats and wastes.
• Get lots of natural carbohydrates from raw fruits and veggies.
• Keep the salt shaker on the table and out of your hands.
• Stay away from extra seasonings and high-fat-content cheeses, especially cellulite's look-alike, cottage cheese.

Avoid: Diuretics, cigarettes, sugar, soft drinks, alcohol, animal fats, chocolate, and fried foods.

Get more exercise. Think not? When was the last time you saw an athlete with dented thighs?

AND HERE'S THE RUB

Friction rubs, from my own experience, work wonders on cottage-cheese thighs. I really like the Method Elancyl™, which is available in drug and department stores nationwide. This French system consists of a hard plastic "mit" with an underside of bumpy rubber. A bar of special soap is placed inside the mit, and you simply massage the affected areas for several minutes each day as you shower or bathe. To complete the routine, there is a special Elancyl cream which is massaged onto the areas after the shower.

And believe me, it's worth a few minutes a day to spend a lifetime without lumpy legs.

OH THOSE ACHES AND VEINS

Gilda Marx, President of Body Designs by Gilda and creator of the Flexatard Leotard, doesn't have one visible dent, vein, or bulge anywhere. Here's her system for easing the aches of veins in your legs: If you're a jogger, become an ex-jogger. Running is not wonderful for varicose or prominent surface veins. As a general rule, prop up your legs every night regardless of how they feel. But when your legs *are* aching, gently massage the areas that ache, then prop your legs on the wall at a 45° angle for about 5 minutes. Or . . . lie on your back and bring your knees up to your chest and then above your head. And be especially diligent about relieving leg stress if varicose veins run in your family. The legs you save may be your own.

CHERYL TIEGS' BOUNCE FOR BUMPS

Do your legs bump where they shouldn't and lump where you wished that they wouldn't? When Cheryl Tiegs, author of *The Way to Natural Beauty*, appeared on the "Good Looks Line," she gave listeners this remedy for saddle bags: Place your legs as far apart as you can without losing your balance. Then turn your toes out. Now

Relieve Those Aches and Veins. If your legs ache, or varicose veins run in the family, be sure to prop your legs up each night, and try bringing your knees to your chest and then over your head.

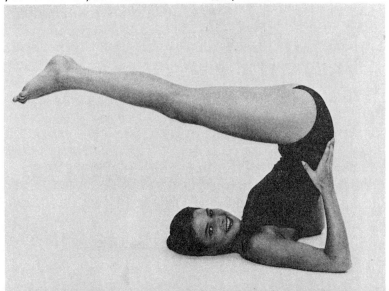

tuck your bottom under and hold your stomach as tightly as you can. Then simply bend your knees as much as you can and bounce up and down without straightening your knees. If you are doing the exercise correctly you will probably feel the inner thighs tightening as you go. Bounce for 1 minute a day to keep the bumps at bay.

Living as Exercise

Cheryl also explained that she makes it a normal part of everyday life to incorporate activity with exercise. For example, every time she drops something on the floor she retrieves it by keeping her legs and knees straight and bending from the waist. It's great for the thighs. But remember, use it to retrieve lost hair clips and books, not stray children weighing over 6 pounds.

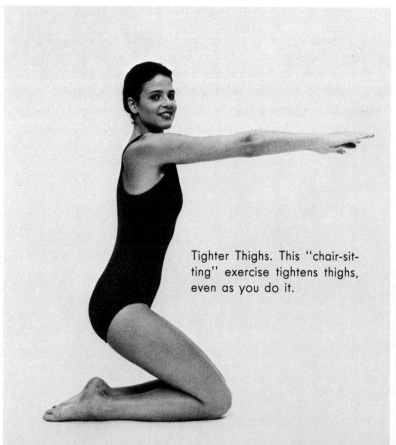

Tighter Thighs. This "chair-sitting" exercise tightens thighs, even as you do it.

THIGH TIGHTENER

Sit on the floor with your feet tucked under you, bottom resting lightly on your heels. Hold your arms out straight at shoulder level, and lift yourself slowly to a chair-sitting position. As you rise, tighten your thigh muscles. Lower yourself slowly and repeat 5 times a day to start, building up, eventually to 20 a day.

SLIMMING IN THE SAND

You don't have to wait for the cows to come home for great calves, if you practice these exercises daily. They work wonders. Next time you're at the beach, dig little holes in the sand by flexing, then curling your toes. And remember, always take advantage of the beach sand for a walk or run. The give of the sand gives you almost double the benefit of a hard surface.

ANOTHER CALF SHAPER

Sit on the edge of a chair and rest your heels on the floor, with your feet parallel and a few inches apart. Flex your foot slowly and point your toes as hard as you can. Now, bring your toes back until they are pointing upward. Repeat 10 times.

BUILDING UP THIN LEGS

The old idiom that you can never be too rich or too thin may be fine for cocktail party chatter, but not if you're the one who's self-conscious because you're too thin. If you feel that your legs can use some shaping up, try this exercise for skinny legs:

Stand straight with toes pointed out, heels together. Hold onto a chair with one hand for support, rise up on your toes, and sink down into a knee bend, staying on your toes and keeping your back straight. Stretch up again and then lower your heels. Repeat 10 times. If you really want to beef up skinny legs, you might consider exercising with leg weights. Try 2 to 5 pounds for starters. A good

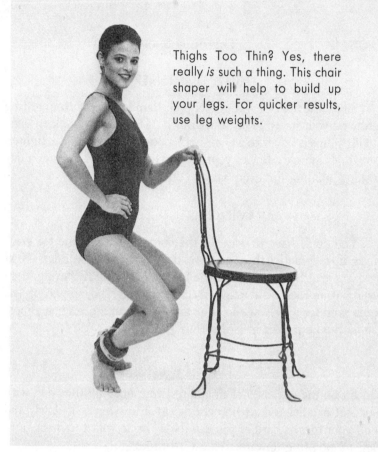

Thighs Too Thin? Yes, there really *is* such a thing. This chair shaper will help to build up your legs. For quicker results, use leg weights.

source for uncomplicated exercises is a nifty illustrated book called *The Complete Encyclopedia of Exercises* by the Diagram Group.

UPPER-ARM FIRMERS, STOMACH TURNERS, AND BETTER HINDSIGHTS

UPPER-ARM FIRMERS

Try incorporating body-revving activities into your normal everyday routines, by using your body in different ways. For example, prop your leg up on the wash basin and stretch it out when you brush your teeth. Or direct it behind you like a ballet dancer, and keep level. Reverse legs and hold. Another trick to get your metabolism in high gear is to put your pantyhose on while lying down on the bed. Remove them in the evening in the same manner. Finally, if you are a frequent subway rider, forget competing for a seat and go for the strap. It's a great upper-arm firmer and circulation mover.

ARM-ER SUITING

Another way to firm your upper arms are flexes. *Here's how:* Sit straight, arms close to your body, elbows bent. Push your elbows back behind you until you feel the stretch in your shoulder blades. Keeping your elbows still, straighten your arms, then return to a bent position. Do 10 times a day.

BETTER HINDSIGHTS

BUTTOCKS' BOUNCE

Want to bounce more than an ounce from your seat? *Try this:* Sit on the floor with your hands at your sides, palms flat on the floor. Then lift from the hips and bounce back to the floor so that part of your hip and part of your buttocks hit the floor with each bounce. Start with about five bounces on the left. Then relax, take a deep breath, and begin five more on the right. Work up to twenty buttocks' bounces a day—to tone up your muscles and tissues.

TUSHY TIGHTENER

While you're lying on your back (or sitting at your desk), simply tighten the buttocks. Hold the position for 5 seconds and release.

STOMACH TURNERS (FROM FAT TO FLAT)

PRESS FOR SUCCESS

If the closest distance between you and the rest of the world is your stomach, you need to exercise to get it flat and tight again. Here's an exercise for keeping your stomach firm that really works!

Ready? Breathe out all of the air in your lungs, now press your stomach with your palms, keeping your elbows at right angles to your body. Continue to breathe deeply, inhaling through your nose and exhaling through your mouth. But keep pressing your stomach as hard as you can with both hands.

SUZY PRUDDEN'S SPARE TIRE DEFLATOR*

- First, stand straight with your feet apart. Shoes off.
- Now, bend forward at the hips, but be sure your back is straight.
- Then, tighten your hands into fists and bend your arms. Your fists should almost meet in front of your chest.
- Next, twist your torso up to the right, keeping your arms in their original position. Your right elbow should point toward the ceiling, your left elbow toward the floor.
- Last, reverse the position of your body, twisting your torso up to the left and raising your left elbow.
- Twist back and forth eight times.
- Warning—to prevent dizziness, look at the floor while you do the twist. Naturally, get the go-ahead signal from your physician before doing this, or any other physical activity.

TUMMY TONER

Sit on the floor with one leg extended in front of you and the other leg bent with your foot flat, so that the heel of your foot is near

---

*From *I Can Exercise Anywhere* (Workman Press) by Suzy Prudden and Jeffrey Sussman.

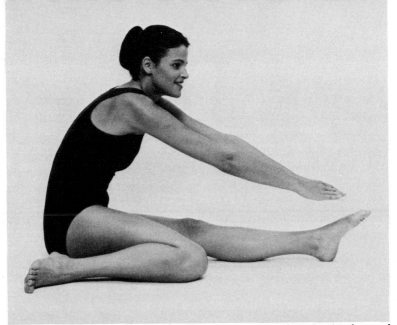

Tummy Toner. To go from fat to flat, force yourself to do this form of sit-up as many times as you can.

the buttock on the same side. Stretch your arms overhead and . . . slowly stretch and bend forward from the hips so that your arms are reaching out toward the extended leg. Then return to your original position and switch to the other leg. Repeat eight times a day for the first week, and, sixteen times a day for the second.

You'll begin to see your tummy get tighter and stronger within the first few weeks of workout. And that's worth struggling for!

BEAUTY AND THE BREAST

THE BREAST TEST

Wondering whether you would, could, or should go braless? Then try these tests which will give you the answers in no time . . . flat.

Stand up straight au naturel. Place a pencil under the breast-fold crease. If the pencil falls toward the floor, chances are your breasts don't, and you are free to go braless whenever the urge hits. If, however, the pencil doesn't budge I would advise that you not burn your bra . . . not yet anyway.

Here's another test: Stand in front of a mirror. Lift your arms, hands up, over your head. If the nipple is higher than the breast-fold crease, your breasts are probably firm enough for you to go without a bra. If not, don't despair, because you'll find some pectoral-firming exercises later on in this chapter.

BREAST FIRMERS AND SHAPERS

If you've failed the previous breast tests, don't despair! It just means that you can use a lift . . . literally. And exercise can help you get it. But remember, breasts are made up of 80 percent glandular tissue and 20 percent fat. Exercise canNOT, repeat, canNOT change the shape of your breasts, but it will help to firm them. These exercises are designed to firm up the pectoral muscles that support the breasts.

THE CLASSIC

Stand with your back straight. Grasp wrists tightly with the opposite hands. Pretend to push your sleeves up without letting your hands slide up your arms. The tension should cause a slight jump in the breast area. Hold to a full count of three. Repeat 10 times.

GILDA MARX'S WAY

Get down on all fours with your palms flat on the floor and directly under your shoulders. Keep your elbows straight and your knees bent. Now, lower your entire body, until your chest touches the floor. Then straighten your arms and come back up again. Now, here's the kicker: While you're doing this exercise, extend one leg behind you and keep it raised to a point no higher than your hips. Repeat the exercise 10 times.

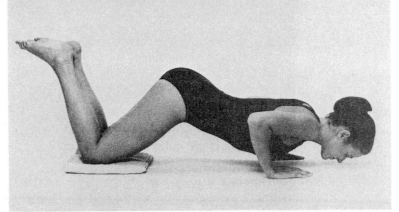

Breast Firmer. While you cannot change the shape or size of your breasts through exercise, you *can* make them firmer and shaplier. This is Gilda Marx's way.

TAKE A COLD SHOWER

Make a habit of taking a cold shower for your breasts after your normal shower. Aim the shower head or hand-held attachment toward your breasts, and run the cold water for about a minute. A cold shower should only be taken by those in perfect health, however, and it's best to check with your doctor. But be sure to avoid hot water altogether as it can contribute to breast droopiness. And, during your bath, use a natural-textured friction mit to stimulate allover circulation.

OTHER DO'S AND DON'TS

• Do apply a rich moisturizer to your breast in circular, inside-to-outside motions each night before you retire.
• Do give your breasts tiny, very delicate pinches with your thumb and forefinger. Pinch upward until the flesh slips out of your fingers. Be gentle and repeat all over your breasts.
• Do swim! And the breaststroke, of course, is the best way to do it.
• Do daily deep-breathing exercises.
• Do exercise the breasts by contracting the large neck muscle 10 to 50 times a day.

• Don't wear bras that are too tight, but do be sure to wear one that fits well for all sports.
• Do use firming lotions and creams designed solely for the breast daily. Clarins products are quite good.
• Don't lose or gain too much weight too quickly.
• Do improve your posture if it isn't good.
• And finally, try this: Lie on your stomach and lift your torso and legs off the ground simultaneously several times a day.

MEASURING UP . . . TO FIND THE RIGHT SIZED BRA

Do you know that wearing the wrong bra size can make you look flat, fat, or just plain droopy? Or that 75 percent of the women in the United States wear the wrong sized bra? If the band rides up in the back, the bra size is too large. If it causes bulges in the front or sides, the bra size or cup size is too small. Here's how to tell what's right for you: Measure yourself underneath your bust, right where the bra band would be. Then add 5 inches to the measurement. That's your bra size. (If you are exceptionally small-boned, add *only* 4 inches.) For example, if you measure 29 and add 5 inches, your bra size should be 34. To find the cup size, measure around the fullest part of your bust. If it measures a half inch over the bra size, you should choose a Double "A" cup. One inch—an "A", 2 inches —a "B", 3 inches—a "C", 4 inches—a "D", and 5 inches—a Double "D." So you see, it's never too late to learn your A,B,Cs!

THE RIGHT BRAS

FOR LARGE BREASTS

The pros at Playtex have discovered that about 35 percent of the women in this country are size 16 and over, which means that 35 percent of all women wear bra sizes over 36. So, going braless is probably just not that desirable to you if you fall into this category. But it doesn't mean that you have to truss yourself like a turkey, either. You *can* look gorgeous, and even more importantly, *feel* comfortable by following these suggestions:

Buy bras that have more coverage in the center front. They should also have straps that are wider and not too stretchy. Test the straps by jumping up and down in the try-on room. Do you bounce more than you'd like? The straps should ideally be made of a rigid type of stretch fabric, or be of non-stretch cloth.

Remember too, that bras with seams will give you more support and shaping, while seamless bras will give you a smooth, natural look. But a bra should fit you perfectly, or you may have too much droop in your scoop neck!

FOR SMALL BREASTS

Do you think of yourself as an under achiever . . . at least where your bustline is concerned? Well, the small-busted woman can look just as provocative as the full-figured woman—*with* the proper bra. While you need less support, you may like a bit of help. For example, try a bra with a little fiberfill when you want to look fuller; a seamless bra, when you want to look softer. Wear a push-up bra when you want to look just plain *sensational* in plunging necklines.

Finally, the only way to know what bra works best for you is to try, before you buy!

FOR AVERAGE BREASTS

Are you average . . . at least as far as your figure is concerned? Lucky you! An average figure means that your body is in proportion. Your bust measurement around the fullest part is from 10 to 12 inches larger than your waistline. Your hips around their fullest part are approximately the same as your bust. Look for seamless styles to go under T-shirts and sweaters, push-up or front-closure bras to wear under plunging necklines, and lacy styles . . . any time!

BREAST SELF-EXAMINATION

Stand as straight as you can. Raise your arm on the side to be examined. Hold your other hand straight with fingers extended and press your palm against the breast. Feel for any lumps, look for any discharge. Repeat the procedure on the other side, with the other arm raised. Standing in front of a mirror, check for depressions, any puckering of the skin, or changes in the shape of the breasts.

Examine your breasts every month, 1 week after your period ends. If you do notice any abnormalities, contact your doctor immediately. Early detection of breast cancer has saved the lives of countless women.

A HOME TEST TO TELL THE DIFFERENCE BETWEEN A PROBLEM LUMP AND A GLAND

If you're familiar with breast self-examination, you may be concerned when you feel a lump that wasn't there before. Dr. Albert Milan, attending obstetrician, and gynecologist at Baltimore's Union Memorial Hospital, and author of *Breast Self-Examination*, devised this test that can help show you the difference between a milk gland, or cyst, and a potentially harmful fixed lump.

Place your fingertip on your closed eyelid. Gently move your eyelid over the eyeball. The eyeball feels slippery and moves. Your lid glides smoothly over it. Next: Pinch your lid, lifting it away from your eyeball. It lifts freely, and easily. Now, place the ball of your fingertip on the end of your nose. Try to move the skin beneath it, without moving your nose tip. It won't move. It's fixed, and, your nose tip moves with your skin. Now, pinch the skin on your nose tip between your fingertips. Try to lift it. You can't. Similarly, a fixed lump won't move, a gland or cyst in the breast will. But, check out *any* breast lump with your doctor.

LOOSENED UP INSTEAD OF UPTIGHT

TENSION-FIGHTING EXERCISES

No time to relax? Well, relaxing is vital to getting the most out of what you eat, and for using energy properly, and for feeling your best. But if, try as you may, there just doesn't seem to be any time to relax try these quick tips:

Joy Gross, Director of The Pawling Health Manor, recommends the following for relaxing the face and neck: Clamp the teeth together and smile widely while tilting the chin upward. Hold for a beat, let go. Repeat.

Another good muscle loosener is the "Head Roll." Again stand relaxed, with your knees straight and your feet apart. Drop your head forward. Slowly roll your head back, as far as you can. At the same time, jut your chin forward, and repeat.

BODY UNTEASER

Concentrate and tense up your entire body . . . and that includes your face. Then release. You'll feel lots better, and lots more relaxed.

MORE TENSION FIGHTERS

NAURA HAYDEN'S BREATHACISE

As you awaken, slowly exhale through your mouth. Keep exhaling until there's not a drop of stale air left. Then hold it for 5 seconds. Slowly inhale through your nose till your lungs feel full, and hold this for a count of 50. Repeat this exercise four times. Believe it or not, by the fifth exhale, your brain will be so alert, it may startle you.

BREATHLESS RELAXER

Sit very still in any straight-backed chair. Keep your feet flat to the floor, tune out your surroundings and inhale through your nose and . . . imagine the breath traveling up your forehead, over your head and back down your spine. As you exhale through your mouth, picture the breath traveling upward just in front of your body. Do about 20 complete "Circle" breaths. While it may sound strange, it really works. You'll feel relaxed, and, ready to go!

ENERGY CRISES RELIEVERS

GILDA MARX'S BED FRAME OF MIND

What's the best thing you can do for yourself in bed? If you guessed what I think you guessed, you're wrong and if you guessed exercise your aches away . . . you're right. Begin tomorrow morning before you even get out of bed.

Bring your arms straight back, part your feet slightly, and stretch and elongate your spine very slowly for about a minute or two. Place your arms at your sides and slide your leg up and down . . . bending your knee . . . for a count of two. Do each leg 10 times at a slow, normal tempo to start. Now, that's a real circulation revver and body energizer. And, believe it or not, *that's* the best thing you can do for your body in bed!

REV UP AT WORK

California fitness star, David Luna, stretches for energy. Do you know how to stretch for success? Stretching your body, especially if you have a job that keeps you desk bound, can sap you of energy and produce tension. Here's how to stretch for success while you're dressed for success at your desk.

Try the overhand stretch; it's the easiest and most natural stretch of all. Clasp your hands in front of you while seated in a chair.

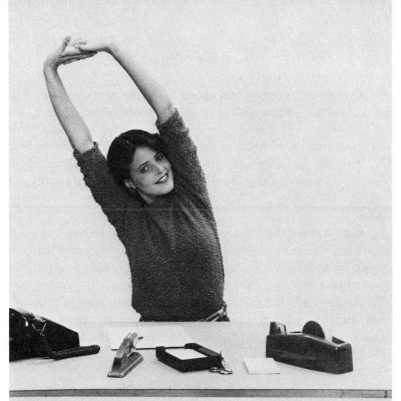

Stretch for Success. Desk-bound and feeling sapped of energy? This overhead stretch can give you an instant power boost.

Keep your fingers together and turn your palms upward toward the ceiling. Straighten your arms over your head. Pull your torso up and bend slightly to the left, then slightly to the right. Hold each position for a few seconds. You can feel the pull through your arms, shoulders, and back, as you feel tensions drain.

RUNNING FOR YOUR LIFE

Think you'd love to get out and run for the health of it? Terrific! But, before you do, you should learn to walk before you jog, and jog before you run . . . running is a wonderful way to shape up your outside, while providing strength for your cardiovascular system, inside.

Orthopedic surgeon and sports medicine physician, Dr. Edward Jones of Greenwich, Connecticut, an expert on the subject, advises a thorough checkup and a stress test before you undertake a running routine. When you get the "all-clear," begin by walking for 2 minutes, then jogging for 2 minutes. Jogging is the easiest, most leisurely form of running. Do this for about 20 minutes, alternating jogging and walking for 2-minute stints. Count time rather than distance.

Give yourself the talk test when you feel tired: Never run when your wind is so short that you can't talk. In time, you'll find that you can jog more, walk less. Eventually, you can incorporate running into your routine. But it takes time to build stamina.

At the start, run on flat surfaces, with your body erect, chin back, arms low and freely flowing. Run on the fore foot as much as possible. Running takes patience. Patience to start slowly, build slowly. Too much too soon is not only an unrealistic goal, it's an unsafe one.

STRETCH FOR SUCCESS

Successful runners begin and end each running session with exercise . . . about 10 minutes before and 5 minutes *after* each run. Stretching your muscles is one of the most important things you can do. Begin with wall push-ups. . . . They are great shaper-uppers. Stand about 18 inches from the wall, with your palms flat to the wall. Lean forward with heels planted firmly, and hold for 10 seconds. Relax. Do this 10 times to stretch the calf and the hamstring muscles.

MORE STRETCH FOR YOUR STEP

To stretch calf muscles and Achilles tendon, stand on a stair edge with heels hanging over. Rise up on the balls of your feet and return back slowly. Don't slam down, you might lose your balance . . . not to mention the race!

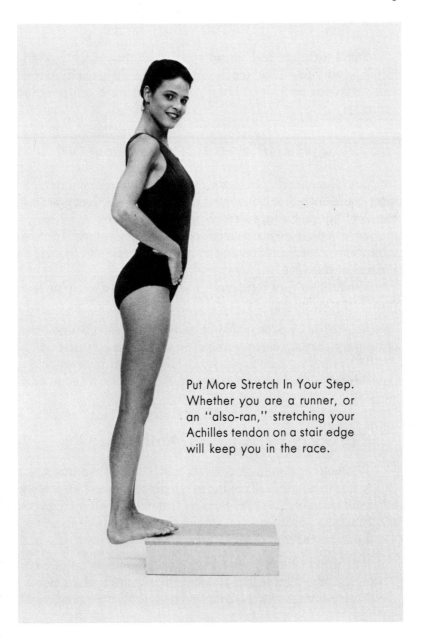

Put More Stretch In Your Step.
Whether you are a runner, or
an "also-ran," stretching your
Achilles tendon on a stair edge
will keep you in the race.

WHEW! STRETCH SOME MORE

Stand with your feet spread apart wider than shoulder width. Slowly bend forward and touch your palms to the ground. As your muscles loosen with time, bring your feet closer together as you stretch.

OUCH! AND WHAT TO DO ABOUT IT

Since running is a percussion exercise, it can cause injuries. The most common preventable ones, according to Dr. Jones, are leg, foot, and hip problems, followed by pulled or strained muscles.

So, if you experience pain in front of your leg—it may be a shin splint. This comes from running on uneven surfaces and running on surfaces of different hardnesses.

What to do? Just rest, apply moist heat, and take aspirin with your doctor's approval.

Bonus Tip: Aspirin should be taken with a full glass of water, or during a meal to decrease the chance of stomach irritation.

When you're ready to run again, be sure to increase stretching exercises before and after each run. And, apply ice to any strained areas.

RUNNING SHOE RECOMMENDATIONS

Running in crummy gym shorts or an old grey sweatsuit won't alter your running style. Running in crummy shoes will. A properly fitted pair of running shoes can mean the difference between success and failure . . . between comfort and agony.

Look for these qualities in a running shoe:

- The heel of the shoe should be twice the thickness of the sole, with the ideal height at about three-quarters of an inch.
- Your running shoes should have a breathable upper, prefera-

bly one of mesh, leather, or nylon . . . plastic doesn't allow for air circulation.

• Look for comfort rather than flashy design . . . *you'll* be wearing the shoes, not the designer. Allow three-quarters of an inch between your toes and the front of the shoe to allow for foot slide.

• Shoes should fit snugly at the heel and have a good arch support.

• Finally, don't trust the kid in the shoe department to understand your needs. Try the shoes on and then, if you've got the nerve, test them by running around the store.

BEAUTY AND THE BEACH

Ever notice how tan becomes more precious than gold in the summer? But it wasn't until the 1920s, when legend says Zelda Fitzgerald bared body and soul to the sun, that sunning became a national pasttime. Before that, a tan was thought to be the weatherbeaten result of neglect . . . something for farmers and sailors only. Now, however, countless millions spend countless hours attempting to turn white into tan and tan into bronze. Unfortunately, you can prematurely age yourself at the least, and develop skin cancer at the worst, with too much of a good thing.

TAN WITHOUT TEARS

Everyone knows by now that too much sun has ruined too much skin, but you might not know that it will take at least 10 years for the damage to show. Sun-damaged skin acts very much the same as skin that is simply aging . . . only it does it much sooner. The cells don't turn over as quickly, the collagen fibers thicken, and other aging factors set in. So you can have leathery prematurely aged skin at 30 or great looking skin at 70. The determining factors are heredity . . . which you can't do a lot about, and sun exposure . . . which you *must* do a lot about.

While all this advice sounds fine for a 15-year-old planning for the future, what if you're 35 or 50 and have been playing tennis or working in the sun all of your life? Well, here's the good news: While you can't reverse the damage that's already been done, you can slow down the rate at which the aging process proceeds in the future!

Unfortunately, skin doesn't come in wrinkle-free fabrics, so you've got to protect it. It *is* possible to get a safe tan, but you have to know *how* to approach the sun.

SKIN CARE EXPERT IRMA SHORRELL'S TAN COMMANDMENTS

• The ultraviolet rays of the sun are usually strongest at midday, so mornings and later afternoons are best for sunning.
• Apply sunscreen at least 45 minutes before you sunbathe and again after swimming or heavy exercise.
• Be careful about your shoulders, knees, nose, lips, tops of feet, and ears. Give them an extra layer of protection. A lip block or a dark opaque lipstick will help protect lips.
• Ultraviolet rays *do* penetrate through overcast clouds, wet T-shirts, and the water. Don't fool yourself into believing you're safe under these conditions.
• Sand and other light surfaces act as sun reflectors and increase your chances of burning up, so take extra care.
• Remember! Wet skin is burned more easily than dry.

THE NUMBERS GAME

Recently, sunscreening products have been developed with numerical ratings called sun protection factors, or SPF. The ratings— from 2 through 15—indicate how much longer you can stay in the sun *with* the product applied than you could without it. Here's how it works: A lotion marked with an SPF of 2 means that you can stay in the sun without getting a burn two times longer than you could without protection. A lotion marked 4 means you can stay four times longer, and so forth.

Ask your doctor which product and which sun protection factor is best for you.

SUNBURN-CAUSING SUBSTANCES

Have you ever spent a day in the sun and found a burn where your cologne used to be? It's probably a photosensitive reaction to the sun. Believe it or not, some colognes and even some foods can cause your skin to become extra sensitive to sunlight.

Here are some culprits:

• Lime, a favorite summer fruit and fragrance, can cause a sunburn. Even a stray lime squirt from a drink can cause a burn where it's landed on your skin.
• Perfumes that contain oil of bergamot can cause this reaction, as can certain foods like carrot and celery extract.
• Some deodorant soaps can be very photosensitizing to your skin. If you use a deodorant soap, don't shower with it before a day in the sun.
• Diuretics, tranquilizers, and acne medicines such as vitamin A acid. If you're using any medications like these, check with your doctor before you hit the beach.

SUNSPOTS

If you react with skin discolorations instead, just give them time to fade. All the scrubbing in the world won't help.

SOOTHING YOUR SUNBURN

Have you done everything you shouldn't and gotten yourself good and sunburned? First of all, you've got to hydrate your skin . . . put back some of the moisture it's lost. Bathing can help. Take a plain bath in lukewarm water. After you've soaked for a while, about 15 or 20 minutes, add your bath oil. This will help to seal in the water that's been absorbed by your skin. If you prefer showers, spray your bath oil onto your skin while you're still wet. Then gently pat dry with a towel.

Always apply a good moisturizer. Once the skin is hydrated, it won't be parched, and this will help prevent peeling. It's really only the dried-out skin that peels off. If you keep to this routine religiously, even after the burn stops burning, you'll not only feel better, but you'll probably prolong the tan you've worked so hard to get.

STRAPPED

If the only time your bathing suit strap marks don't show . . . is when you're wearing the suit itself, not to worry! You don't have to live with stripes all summer. Here's what to do: Just cover any blank spaces with a quick tanning cream such at QT™ from Coppertone, and in a few hours, the proteins in your skin will react to the tanning ingredients in the cream, so that nontanned areas will blend in with the rest of you.

PARTING THOUGHTS

Are you protecting every part of you from the sun? You're not if you forget the part in your hair. But, don't think you have to slop on globs of sunscreen. All you need is a sunscreen stick. It's much neater and just as effective. Just streak it onto the part in your hair 45 minutes before sun exposure.

Remember too, if you pull your hair up while sunning, or even just strolling, don't forget to sunscreen the nape of your neck.

BEAUTY AND THE BATH

Do you love to spend long hours soaking in a steaming hot tub? If you do, you are probably doing yourself more harm than good.

Water that is too hot can actually dry your skin. The higher the water temperature, the more quickly natural body moisture evaporates as you cool off and moisture is what keeps your skin soft and supple.

For a super moisturizing bath, fill the tub with plain lukewarm water. While the tub is filling, place a big fluffy towel on the radiator to heat up. Get in the tub and soak for about 20 minutes. This will give your skin the time it needs to absorb sufficient moisture. *Then* pour in your favorite bath oil and soak for an additional 5 minutes. Your bath oil will lie on top of your skin, locking in the water that has already been absorbed.

If you prefer showers, dab or massage your bath oil onto your skin while you're still wet. This is a good routine to get into daily.

When drying off, pat gently with the heated towel. AAAAh, spa!

WAYS AND WAYS OF SOAKING IT UP

INSTANT NONFAT MILK BATH

Fill the tub with warm water and pour a package of dry milk into the tub under the running water. Swish it around to dissolve the milk completely. Step in and just relax. A milk bath without the cholesterol—which will also help to soothe your sunburn.

If you're out of dry milk you can do the same thing by pouring a quart of regular low-fat milk into the tub. But this practice is a lot more expensive and probably not as much fun.

LUXURY SPA BATH FOR PENNIES

First, begin by collecting as many little sample vials of perfume as you can. In fact, make it a point to ask for free samples every time you go into a department store. Then whenever the urge to splurge on a perfumed bath hits, just pour a vial or two of perfume and a couple of capfuls of baby oil into a warm . . . not hot . . . bath. Sit back and pretend that you are on the French Riviera.

FATIGUE-FIGHTING VINEGAR BATH

An apple-cider vinegar bath can help you to overcome fatigue, detoxify certain elements in your skin, help relieve itchiness, even help soothe poison ivy and sunburn. Just add two cups of apple-cider vinegar to your warm bath water, before you add yourself.

Apple-cider vinegar can be used too, as a bath splash and fatigue-fighter, by splashing some onto your shoulders, arms, back, and chest.

MADEMOISELLE'S PERSONALIZED BATHS

Take 2 tablespoons of rosemary, 2 tablespoons of chamomile, and 1 sprig of fresh chopped mint. Tie the mixture up in a little muslin or cheesecloth bag . . . just like bouquet garni. Then hold it under the tap as the tub fills.

If you love bubble baths on the other hand, but yours is all gone, head for the laundry room. Not to bathe, but to borrow. A handful of soap powder, the gentle kind that you use for lingerie, makes an instant fragrant bubble bath.

A FACIAL FOR YOUR BODY

Next time you shower or bathe, try this: While you're still wet, rub a small amount of petroleum jelly into the palms of your hands. Then smooth it all over your body, from head to toe. Replenish with more petroleum jelly as needed.

TWO-FORS

This one is from Gloria Gaynor. Spray some unscented cocoa-butter body lotion with your favorite fragrance. Then smooth it all over your body after you bathe. Not only will you smell wonderful, and feel wickedly delightful, but the treatment won't clash with your other fragrance, nor will it break your bank.

Bonus Tip: Apply extra to the back of your hands. It's a delightful surprise when someone's clever enough to kiss you there. On the practical side? It's a great way to conserve your best fragrance.

WOMEN HAVE THE RIGHT TO BARE ARMS . . . AND LEGS

DEFUZZING WITHOUT TEARS

If the thought of defuzzing is enough to make you cover up again, don't. There's more than one way to skin a cat, or shave a lady.

If you want a really smooth shave, and a moisturizing treat to boot, try baby oil or your favorite bath oil instead of shaving cream. Next time you shower, rub your legs generously with oil, then shave and rinse. But, please be sure to stand on a rubber bath mat to prevent slipping.

- If shaving's not your thing, try waxing. The only problem is that you should have a full 3 weeks' growth of hair before you can wax or be waxed effectively. If that involves your legs, be prepared to live in pants while the hair grows in.
- Another effective method is depilatory creams and lotions. These products break down the protein in the hair and dissolve it under the skin. Be sure to do a patch test first, as with any new product.
- The final popular method of dealing with unwanted hair is cream bleach. While it doesn't remove the hair, it does lighten it, almost to the point of invisibility.

SHAVE LADY?

Had too many close shaves lately? If your legs look like you're wearing polka-dotted pants after shaving, you're probably shaving too closely, in the wrong direction. The latest word is that shaving *against* the grain may cause hairs to become trapped inside the skin and this can lead to folliculitis, an inflammation of the hair follicles.

To prevent skin irritation, avoid abrasive sponges after shaving, waxing, or sunburning your legs. And wait at least a day after waxing before playing sports or sunning. Excess perspiration can cause freshly waxed legs to become irritated. Too much sun on unprotected legs can cause permanent damage in the form of spider veins.

SCENT SENSE

Fragrance has been used since the beginning of time to seduce, and even reduce the strongest of souls to the sweetest of romantics. If you'd like to know why, when, and how you should use your fragrance, read on. These tips, which were gathered by The Fragrance Foundation, will help you make the most not only of your scent sense but of your dollars and cents as well.

Did you know that:

• Your sense of smell is not as strong in the morning as the evening? So apply scent more liberally in the morning and more sparingly at night.

• If you are over 50, you may not smell fragrance as strongly? So keep a lighter touch with a fragrance if you are fifty or over. If you are with someone of that age, apply your fragrance more heavily.

• Perfume is the most concentrated form of fragrance, followed by toilet water and then cologne?

• Hot weather calls for lighter scents because heat intensifies fragrance? The opposite, of course, applies to winter.

• Fragrance should be tested directly on your skin? Sniffing a fragrance bottle can't let you know what the fragrance will smell like when it mixes with your own body oils and chemistry.

• Diogenes believed that fragrance rises, and he was right? So consider applying fragrance to your feet as well as your body's pulse and friction spots.

• The best places to apply fragrance are the temples, behind the knees, in the elbow creases and the hollow at the base of the throat, as well as inside the ankles and between the breasts?

• If your skin is oily, you can get away with a scantier application of fragrance? If it's dry you'll need more.

• You should apply a bit before bed? Although your sight sense shuts down during sleep, your scent sense never sleeps.

MALE E-SCENT-IALS

Cologne is the most concentrated form of men's fragrance followed by after-shave lotion (which is less concentrated, and may contain an astringent to help heal nicks and cuts). After-shave may also contain a moisturizer which can help to soften the skin, especially when it is applied while the skin is still moist.

SCENT CENTS

If you've ever bought an expensive bottle of perfume, cologne, or after-shave and discovered after you've gotten it home that it just wasn't "you," it will help if you remember:

• The myriad of scents in the store can be confusing to your nose. After you've tested fragrance on your skin, give it time to blend with your personal body chemistry. And don't attempt to try more than three fragrances at once.

• Use toilet water, which uses the same essences as perfumes, as a base for perfume once you've found one you love.

• You should always shield your fragrances from temperature extremes because exposure can upset the chemical balance.

• It's not a good idea to hoard your favorite fragrance for a special day, as scents left too long in a bottle can spoil or even evaporate.

• Remember that each fragrance smells different on each person. Choose your fragrance because you love the way it smells on *you.*

WONDERFUL MISCELLANEOUS BODY AND MIND FACTS

GOOD LOVIN' CAN HELP KEEP YOU HEALTHY

It may interest you to know, that love, like water, is good for you, especially when you're in it. A research project has recently shown that when a group of rabbits (who are notoriously famous for being in love) were held, talked to, played with, and petted on a regular basis their cholesterol buildup was reduced. The control group, the bunnies who got no loving at all and were even ignored a lot, developed fatty plaques in their coronary arteries. And that points up something very significant: We do, in fact, need love . . . the kind you fall into, are born into, and mature with. Remember, love can make you healthy. And when you marry well, even wealthy. It will not, however, ever make you wise!

GOOD FRIENDS EQUAL GOOD HEALTH, TOO

Good friends are also medically good for you. A recent survey at Yale showed that the more friends, relatives, and social contacts a person has, the less likely that person is to die of illness or in an accident! In fact, a person without a solid network of close friends is 2.8 times more likely to have a shorter life than those who are solidly connected. (That's the loving kind of social connection, not the social-climbing kind.) In fact, social climbing has been known to kill many people before their time, possibly from eating too many hors d'oeuvres on the ladder to upward mobility. In any case, the survey pointed up that there can be damaging chemical changes when one lacks human companionship. So if you don't have any, get some. The life you extend may be your own.

FLYING FACTS

Traveling across time zones can interfere with the way your body functions, especially after long flights. To prevent major interferences, you should adopt a new wake/sleep pattern, thus adjusting your internal body clock. For example, if you're traveling west, try going to bed an hour later than usual and getting up an hour earlier, for several days before departure. Traveling east? The opposite applies. This will help you to avoid jet lag . . . and eye bag!

FLYING UNHIGH

Another way to avoid unpleasant body crazies when flying is to avoid sleeping pills, cigarettes, and alcohol. For example, cigarette smoke contains carbon monoxide which reduces the blood's ability to carry oxygen. Sleeping pills confuse the body's time clock and aggravate the problem of jet lag (especially if you are traveling across time zones). And alcohol? It dehydrates the system causing further distortion through jet lag.

Bonus Travel Tip: If you've ever noticed that long trips tend to make your feet swell, it's because the bloodflow is constricted from your feet. So avoid tight clothing, such as second-skin jeans and tight undergarments. If you are flying, riding in a bus, or on a train, get up and move around at least every half hour, and move your feet around every 15 minutes or so.

PREGNANCY AND FLYING

Women in the final trimester of pregnancy may be surprised to learn that air travel should be restricted during this part of the pregnancy. Gravity and air pressure changes have been known, in fact, to induce early labor. So check with a doctor and the airline beforehand. Some airlines even require a doctor's certificate. If you must fly, make it more comfortable for yourself, by requesting that you be allowed to keep your seat semireclined during takeoff. This will help to direct the acceleration pressure upward. To take the strain off of your back muscles, place a few small pillows at the small of your back. And finally, avoid gum and carbonated beverages. Keep these tips in mind while *you* are airborne, or you might end up with an airborne newborn!

BACK ACHES, SEEDS FOR THE WEED, REST FOR THE WEARY

OH MY ACHING BACK!

Low-back pain just might be *the* ache of the '80s. Everyone seems to have it. Its cause? According to Dr. Edward Jones, there are many causes including obesity, a too sedentary life style, weakening of the back and abdominal muscles, and poor posture. But here's the good news: Dr. Jones suggests that much low-back pain can be relieved simply by changing the way in which you move, relax, and exercise. For example, don't ever lift with your arms fully extended; rather bring the object as close to your body as possible. And exercises such as swimming, pelvic tilts, knee to chest, and sit-ups all strengthen back and abdominal muscles.

If, however, the most you ever lift are the dishes at the sink or your elbow at the pub, you might still be causing back aches, simply by standing incorrectly. Any activity, in fact, that requires prolonged standing, should be done with one leg slightly lifted . . . a low footstool at the sink, or the bar rail at your favorite watering hole!

UP IN SMOKE

Have all your attempts to quite smoking gone up in smoke? Well, help may be just a sunflower seed or two dozen away. Sunflower-seed oil tends to cause a bodily reaction similar to smoking. So the substitution of sunflower seeds when the urge to light up hits may be the answer you've been searching for. Simply go out and buy a few pounds of raw, unshelled sunflower seeds. Stash several ounces in pocket or purse, and pop a few in your mouth each time the seedy weedy urges strike. The sooner you start, the sooner you may become an ex-smoker!

SLEEP-INDUCING FOODS

A long, lazy after-dinner nap seems to be part of everyone's Thanksgiving and Christmas traditions. Ever wonder why? Well, it may not be the holiday excitement that tires you out, it may be the turkey you've eaten. Turkey, you see, contains L-tryptophan—an amino acid that is a natural sleep-inducer. So if you're planning to dine on turkey with someone you want to impress, you might decide to have a steak instead. After all, you don't want to fall asleep with your head in the mashed potatoes.

But if sleep is the thing you crave most and do least, try tapping foods with L-tryptophan for natural sleep. Some of the best sources are milk (yes, as in a nice warm glass of before bed), bananas, figs, pineapples, and nuts. And unlike sleeping drugs, tryptophan does not alter normal sleep habits, nor is it accompanied by a sleep hangover.

4
Hand and Foot Notes

Everything That You Could Possibly Ever Want To Do To Your Hands and Feet—Almost.

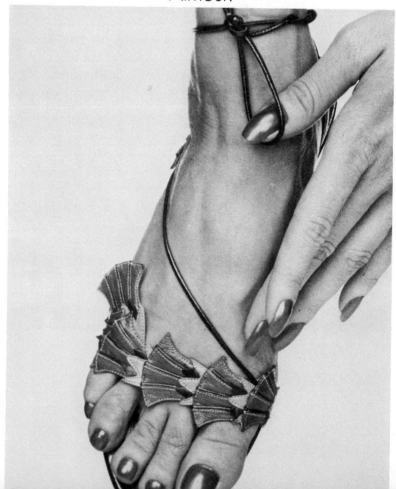

A SHOW OF HANDS

NAIL TALES

Heard any good nail tales lately? How about the one that says that gelatin is great for your nails? According to recent evidence that is one *whale* of a nail tale. Gelatin may not, in fact, do any good at all, but a diet rich in protein does. And finally remember, building nails takes a while, because they grow at the rate of only about an eighth of an inch a month and they do grow slower in winter than they do in summer.

WHITE IODINE . . . NOT BLACK MAGIC FOR HARDER NAILS

What about nail hardeners? Do they work? For some people they do, but for others, the formaldyhyde in the product causes an adverse reaction. So it's best to test the product out for a week or so, on one nail only.

But, here's a tip worth a fortune, that literally costs a few cents: White iodine, a product you'll find in mom and pop type drugstores (not sexy cosmetic counters), will harden nails like crazy. What white iodine does is to discourage flaking and peeling. It hardens the nails and, unlike formaldehyde (the major ingredient in most nail hardeners), it produces very few disagreeable reactions.

To use white iodine, first ask your druggist for some—it won't be displayed, believe me. Then simply apply a bit to each polishfree nail before bedtime, for about a week. After that, you will need to apply the product once a week or so. If you use it too often your nails will become *too* hard and brittle!

Tip: Be sure to stay away from peroxide when using white iodine, however. A surgeon friend of mine was using white iodine to harden his nails (and loving the reaction), when he unfortunately, dipped his fingers in peroxide one day and his nails turned orange.

MOISTURIZING YOUR NAILS

Try massaging baby oil or petroleum jelly directly onto the dry cuticles and nails to strengthen and stimulate circulation and growth.

MANICURE MAGIC

Would you like to have hands that look as though they've never done a bit of work? Then you've got to work at it! Here's how to give yourself an at-home manicure:

- Remove old polish.
- Warm your hand cream vigorously between the palms of your hands to soften it.
- Massage hands, arms, and elbows, concentrating on the fingers and cuticles.
- File the nails evenly, avoiding a too angular look, which can weaken the nail sides. A gently rounded top is best.
- Dip nails into a mild solution of soap and water.
- If your cuticles have never been cut, don't start now. Instead, push cuticles back with a pumice stick, or orange-wood stick wrapped in cotton.
- Use nail polish remover to take off the remaining moisturizer.
- Apply a clear base coat, two coats of color, and a sealing coat.

Bonus Tip: Whether you do it yourself or have a professional manicure, keep the color from chipping by applying a coat of sealer over and just around the underside of the nails the next day, and again the day after that.

THE HAND IS QUICKER THAN THE DRY

Want your nail polish to dry in a flash? Apply a dot of safflower or other vegetable oil to your nails a few minutes after you've finished your manicure. Or dip them gently into a bowl of ice water.

GREASING YOUR PALM

If your hands look as though you've been through hand-to-hand combat, they deserve extra care. Give your hands this overnight treat: Slather a thick coating of Vaseline™, or any petroleum jelly, over and around your hands, and cover them with a pair of thick cotton gloves, before going to sleep. In the morning your hands will be softer, smoother, and ready for some serious holding.

HANGNAIL HANGUP

Do you have a problem with hangnails, or do you have a problem growing *any* nails, hung or not? *Try:*

- A coating of Liquid Nail Patch™ before coloring and then bond the flaking bits together with a drop of Super Glue™.
- Adelaide Farah, of *Health* magazine, also recommends that cutting cuticles can result in hangnails, as can biting, and picking at them, so if you do, *don't.*
- Brittleness and splitting? It may mean poor eating habits. Try more protein, and daily moisturizing.
- Wavy ridges? It may be caused by an illness such as the flu, so soak your unpolished nails in warmed olive oil for 5 minutes a day, followed by a cuticle and nail moisturizer. Buff till a dull sheen appears.
- White spots before your eyes? Don't despair. Addy says that white spots on your nails are caused by bruises and air bubbles in the nail body and will disappear as the nail grows.
- Your nails shouldn't be too hard, either. They should be naturally flexible. So if a product makes your nails too rigid, it

may be splitsville again. Your nails just aren't "breathing." To strengthen the nail "matrix," or growth center, go naked . . . at least on your nails, by removing all polish every few weeks, for a week or so, to give them a breath of fresh air.

• Nicotine stains? Clean your nails with a cotton swab dipped in 20-volume peroxide. Apply it to the nail surface and leave it on for 10 minutes. Rinse well with water and moisturizer. *Remember that this tip is not for you if you are using white iodine for hardening.*

HELP FOR DRY HANDS

Health magazine offers these suggestions to keep your hands moisturized and soft, especially during winter months:

• Protect your hands by using rubber gloves with cotton linings. But remember that hands perspire in gloves, so don't wear them for more than 10 minutes at a time. Perspiration only aggravates dry-skin problems.

• An annoying rash on the hands? It might be what's known as "housewife's dermatitis," caused by overexposure to cold and irritating chemicals. So if you've been working with detergents, wash your hands in lukewarm water to remove all traces of the irritant. Then pat dry and apply a lubricating cream or moisturizer.

• If your hands get dry and chapped, no matter what the season or what the reason, keep hand lotion nearby during the day, so you can reapply it after washing, working, at the office or doing household chores.

HAND SCAN: A BUNCH OF THINGS THAT YOU MAY NOT KNOW ABOUT YOUR HANDS

• Over 70 percent of viruses, are transmitted by hand, according to a recent survey, and not transmitted by germs released in sneezing and coughing. So what do you do if you are about to close the deal of your life and your client, who happens to be sneezing, hacking, and coughing, wants to shake on it? Lose the deal, or wash your hands immediately, if not sooner.

• Looking for something to give you a lift? Give your hands a facial. *Here's how:* Take a moisturizing facial mask and following the package directions for your face, use it on your hands, instead. The brush on/peel off kind are terrific for this. Follow up with a moisturizer.

• Housemaid's elbow? If you remember that little ditty from childhood about "Mable, Mable, keep those elbows off the table," try to remember it now that you've grown up. Keeping your elbows on the table, the desk, even the arm of an unpadded chair can result in rough, red, dried-out elbows. To correct it, soak in a tub for minutes with your elbows submerged. Rub a wet cake of peanut-oil soap against those areas. Follow up with an emollient moisturizer.

Note: Yes, I know an elbow isn't really a part of your hands, but it's closer to your hands than to your feet.

FOOT NOTES

PEDICURE LIKE A PRO

I must say, straight out and honest that there are only two things that I can think of that feel quite as wonderful as a professional pedicure. And one of them *is* a professional pedicure. I do believe that everyone should indulge in a quick pro ped at least a few times a year.

But, truth be told, pro pedicures are expensive, and, aside from the loveliness of it, there is really no reason that you can't get the same results at home. *Here's how:*

- Remove all old polish with nail polish remover and soak your feet in a basin of hot soapy water. Clairol's Foot Fixer™ is wonderful for this. It massages your feet, and heats up the water while you soak. But plain bowl, or Foot Fixer™, let your feet soak for about 5 minutes.
- Pat your feet till almost dry and rub a pumice stone around the underside, concentrating on the heels and balls of each foot.
- Cut a lemon in half and squeeze the juice onto each nail to bleach out discoloration. The two halves can then be cupped around the heel and sole of each foot for 15 minutes for extra softening.
- Massage in moisturizer all around the feet and up the legs, kneading each toe individually.
- File the nails to a squarish shape to avoid ingrown nails.
- Remove excess moisturizer with nail polish remover.
- Separate your toes by folding a tissue lengthwise to about an inch wide. Pull the tissue over and around each toe.
- Apply a clear coat of glaze to protect nail coloration.
- Apply two coats of polish.
- Apply an overcoat for sealing.
- To speed up drying, use a drop of safflower oil, a polish smudge-proofer, or dip your toes into ice water.
- To keep your pedicure gorgeous, apply a second coat of sealer to each nail the next day and again the day after that.

BODY AND SOLE

If all of those gorgeous bodies jogging around the block make you want to get out and get gorgeous yourself, remember your feet first. Sore feet can put you out of commission very quickly, and a few minutes spent on foot care may save you aggravation at the least and athlete's foot at the worst. Here's a checklist:

• Carry an extra pair of sweatsocks and change as needed. Perspiration adds to the moist environment that can make a fungus feel at home.

• Use a powder without starch on your feet and in your shoes. Starch is actually a nutrient that bacteria thrive on and when you use it, you are ringing their dinner bell! ZeaSorb™ Powder is a good one to try.

• Wear bathing sandals when showering in a public facility.

REV UP YOUR FEET TO REV UP YOUR BODY

Ever notice that when your feet are tired, so is the rest of you? Next time your feet say no and your brain says disco, try this:

• Sit on the edge of the bathtub. Run the cold water over and around your feet for one full minute. Then switch to moderately hot water for 1 minute and back again to cold. Alternate running cold and hot water for 5 minutes, finishing up with cold.

• Dry your feet and powder them.

• Lie flat on the floor and prop your legs up on the wall with your arms at your sides. Relax this way for 5 minutes.

You'll feel wonderful, and for sure, your feet won't fail you now!

HOW TO FIX YOUR FEET PROFESSIONALLY IN ONE DAY

If you've tried going West, and found to your horror that you couldn't because your feet hurt too much in your cowboy boots, that may be because your feet are prone to problems.

According to top New York podiatrist, Dr. Louis Shure, Western boots and even high-fashion shoes can cause extreme pain if you're prone to corns, calluses, bunions, or hammer toes.

Until a few years ago, the surgery one would have to go through took a hospital stay, and a month's worth of recovery time. But now, a podiatrist foot surgeon (certified and with the proper facilities) can perform the surgery right in the office in 15 minutes. The microsurgical incision is so tiny that there is very slight pain. And instead of being off your feet for a month or more, you can get back to work the very next day. The correction is permanent, and you can finally wear those fashionable shoes . . . or boots to your heart or foot's content.

GIVING YOURSELF THE BOOT

Boots should, of course, be more than just stylish; they should be comfortable at the least, and supportive at best. Next time you go out to buy boots, look for:

- Ample wiggling room for toes, especially in leather boots.
- A moderate heel height. Heels which are too high can cause pressure to be put on the Achilles tendon.
- Rubber boots are great for snow and rain, but not for a day in the office. Rubber doesn't allow the foot to breath, and if you keep them on all day, no one else will be able to breathe when you take them off.
- Mid-calf boots? Keep cuffs, elastic, and drawstrings loose to prevent circulation problems.

LIBERATE YOUR FEET

How liberated are your feet? Many people, women in particular, are conditioned to tolerate pain as the high price we'll pay for high-priced shoes. Believe me, one of the hardest professional models to find is a good foot model. After spending too many hours in $1,000 shoes, these models develop all kinds of strange looking things on their feet and toes. To prevent strange looking things from growing on your feet remember to:

- Play musical feet. That means changing shoes and heel heights daily.
- Shop for shoes in the afternoon when your feet have expanded to their maximum size.

• Try both shoes on and give them a good test in the store.
• Always buy for the larger foot.
• Make sure that there's about a half inch or so, for toe room, and enough width for the foot to spread with each step.

Before We Say Goodbye

Now that you know how to make up, make out and make it right, there's one more thing that you should know: Make it fun!

Approach the way you look with the same enthusiasm that you approach anything you enjoy. Don't make a career of it . . . just know that with a little time, a lot of patience, and everyone's secrets which you've just discovered in this book, you can't miss.

But, as every beauty authority knows, mistakes are part and parcel of experimenting with—and finding out—what is right for *you*. And remember, a mistake is *not* a forever calamity. Learn to chalk it up and laugh it off, because with any luck it will grow back, or at least it can be removed with baby oil. If it doesn't grow back or come off, you can always dye it a different color!

Seriously, though, 99% of looking like a million is feeling like it. You remember the girl in high school who was not a great beauty, but believed that she was. And by the time you graduated, you probably believed that she was too. What you believe, *can be*. I remember looking at photographs of myself at twelve and deciding that my parents should have been canonized for not only keeping me as long as they did, but liking me besides. I decided, right there and then, that I could live in ankle socks, health shoes and frizzy hair forever, or I could make myself a bit better. And so I tried. And I keep on trying, and I keep on having fun.

Sure, along the way, I managed to turn a natural grey streak in my hair to something resembling Crayola puce, and have managed to get made over into something resembling Charles Bronson, but I did learn something worth knowing: When I look the way which is most comfortable to me, I feel terrific!

Trust me. Feel good about yourself, and know one will ever tell your blind date what a nice personality you have. Ever again.

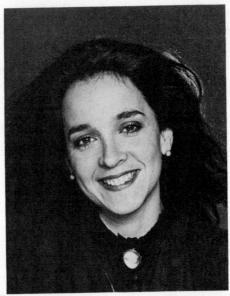

LINDA STASI was creator and host of the popular "Good Looks" daily "Dial-It" program for the telephone company; creator of "Seventeen at School" for *Seventeen* magazine; Beauty & Fashion Editor, *Weight Watchers Magazine*, as well as beauty consultant to dozens of top skin care and cosmetic companies. She lives in New York City.